More praise for
FIRST, DO NO HARM:

"Compelling . . . Solid journalism, packed with vivid, detailed reporting and enough drama to sustain a season of 'St. Elsewhere' episodes."
—*The Boston Globe*

"A cogent presentation of one of our society's most urgent questions: of those who get sick, who will live, and who must be allowed to die? . . . Skillfully and sympathetically woven."
—*The New Yorker*

"Portraits of hospital staff, patients and care-givers include images not easily forgotten: a father saying good-bye to his soon-to-die infant son and a terminally ill teenager writing in crayon, 'Leave me alone,' as his mother talks to him about death."
—*Publishers Weekly*

"Compelling . . . Lisa Belkin properly frames an important national debate on medical ethics."
—*Detroit Free Press*

FIRST, DO NO HARM

Lisa Belkin

BALLANTINE BOOKS • NEW YORK

A Fawcett Book
Published by The Random House Publishing Group
Copyright © 1993 by Lisa Belkin

Published in the United States by Fawcett Books, an imprint of The Random House Publishing Group, a division of Random House, Inc., New York, and distributed in Canada by Random House of Canada Limited, Toronto.

FAWCETT is a registered trademark and the Fawcett colophon is a trademark of Random House, Inc.

www.ballantinebooks.com

ISBN 0-449-22290-X

This edition published by arrangement with Simon & Schuster, Inc.

Manufactured in the United States of America

First Ballantine Books Edition: April 1994

OPM 29 28 27 26 25 24 23

To Bruce,

to Evan, and

to Grandma Pearl

CONTENTS

The physician must be able to tell the antecedents, know the present, and foretell the future—must mediate these things, and have two special objects in view with regard to diseases, mainly, to do good or to do no harm.

—HIPPOCRATES
OF THE EPIDEMICS

MAY

The Committee

It was standing room only in Room 3485 the day the committee voted to let Patrick die.

Nearly three dozen people crammed the small windowless room, outnumbering the two dozen thinly padded chairs. After the seats were filled, latecomers propped themselves against the walls, careful to keep their distance from the dusty chalkboard. Whether sitting or standing, everyone was fidgeting. The emerald carpet only partly silenced the shifting and tapping of their feet.

Lin Weeks's secretary, Ellen Nuñez, always thinks herself lucky when she can book the committee into Room 3485. In Room 4487, the classroom one floor up, the blue-gray carpet is pocked with cigarette burns. Too seedy for her boss's pet committee. Room 5488, one floor higher still, is often reserved for CPR training, and its yellow-white stains, the ghosts of former puddles, are from the Clorox used to disinfect the mannequins' mouths. Too seedy and too depressing. But in this room, Ellen thinks, the varied greens of the carpet, chairs, and chalkboard are calming, or as calm as one can ask for in a hospital. And some pretense of calm is important for these meetings about life and death.

Any soothing effect of the decor, however, was lost on Dr. Javier Aceves, the young pediatrician struggling with Patrick's case. He sat at one end of the long wooden table, with his back to the door and his tired eyes scanning the audience of committee members. Following procedure, he began the session by reciting the basic facts, speaking in the shorthand monotone that is expected at meetings in hospitals.

"Patrick Dismuke is a fifteen-year-old boy, well known to this committee, who is currently in the pediatric critical care unit on a ventilator," he said. "His current hospitalization began two months ago, and this is his second prolonged hospitalization this year . . ."

He needn't have bothered. Everyone in the room knew Patrick. In fact everyone at Hermann Hospital knew Patrick. He had been a patient there for all of his fifteen years, and during that time he spent more days in the hospital than out of it. He had been operated on at least twenty times, probably more, but somewhere along the way his doctors lost count. Although each operation lengthened his life, none came close to curing him.

Patrick was born with Hirschsprung's disease, a disorder of the digestive tract, and after years of surgery to snip out parts of his intestine, he was left unable to digest his food. His was a severe case, and his life was hanging by a literal thread—a thin tube that dripped nutrients and medicines into his veins while he slept. Like most invasions of the body, this one wasn't perfect: He needed the line to live, but the line itself could kill him. Because it broke the barrier between blood and air, it was a bacteria-laden Trojan horse, opening the door to infection and allowing it to overwhelm his body. In turn, the fight against the bacteria caused as many problems as it solved. The constant use of antibiotics provided ideal breeding ground for yeast and other types of fungi.

During the pauses between infections, the veins that

held Patrick's lines would become irritated to the point of collapse, until all the easily reached ones were useless to him. When tubes couldn't be threaded from outside, surgeons opened him up and threaded them from inside. During the last operation the plastic tube was stitched directly into his heart.

Through all this, Patrick was making history. Not the front page headline kind (although, never the shy one, he would have liked that), but the type of news that fills the 20,000 medical journals published worldwide every year. His IV nutrients weren't meant to feed anyone for more than a short period of time, certainly not for fifteen years, and, as far as anyone knew, this was as long as anyone had lived on the milky yellow contents of the squishy plastic sacks. As Javier put it: "We're winging it one day at a time."

The question before the committee was how many more days to wing it. As they spoke, Patrick was upstairs on a ventilator suffering from pneumonia, with a tube down his throat to help him breathe. He was conscious, and he was miserable. His feeding line was working in fits and starts, clogged by infection. He was being simultaneously kept alive and tortured by a nightmare of an antifungal drug called amphotericin B. Over the years, patients unlucky enough to use the drug have renamed it Amphoterrible, or Shake and Bake. The ampho causes violent fevers, which in turn cause chattering chills. It also tends to linger in the kidneys, eating away at the tissue.

For both these reasons doctors don't use the drug a day longer than it takes to kill the infection. Three weeks is considered tolerable, six weeks is of concern, twelve weeks is really too long, but the alternative—free rein for the infection—is still worse than the attempt at a cure. By the time this committee meeting was called, Patrick had been on ampho for eighteen months.

"He'll need a new line soon," Javier said near the end of his little speech. "We know he'll need another one after that and another one after that. Do we keep opening his chest over and over? Without the new line he'll starve. Which is worse?"

He looked up from his notes, folded his hands, and waited for an answer.

Medicine, specifically hospital medicine, is about meetings. Many are as unscheduled and unstructured as doctors gathering with a patient's family in the hallway to get their consent for surgery. Others are more official but stop short of requiring seats—morning rounds, for instance, where the staff walks from bed to bed to bed, allowing those who were on call all night to update those who were at home asleep.

And then there are the full-blown meetings, with membership and agendas and chairmen. It is a telling measure of bureaucracy and economics at Hermann that as many as half its beds are sometimes empty but its conference rooms are often double-booked. Even as the committee decided on the fate of Patrick, another group milled outside, waiting to use the room. Every so often someone at Hermann tries to make a master list of committees and gives up, stymied by the fact that few administrators can remember all the meetings they attend. There was talk several years ago of starting a Committee on Committees to whittle down the number, but that was one group that was never formed. It probably would have been lost, anyway, a lone time slot on a cluttered calender.

There are ever more meetings because there are ever more decisions, and many of them are choices that no human being, with or without a medical degree, should be asked to make. Time was when medicine could do very little for critically ill or dying patients. Now it can do too much. Where to draw the line is the subject of a broad, heated debate throughout the country, a debate that becomes louder with each new medical miracle or impossible case: Should a Michigan doctor be allowed to hook desperate patients to a "suicide machine"? Should the state of Oregon be permitted to deny expensive organ transplants to the poor? Should a fertilized egg, in deep freeze in a laboratory in Tennessee, be considered a "child"? If so, who gets custody when Mom and Dad divorce? Should a Florida man be sent to prison for helping his disease-ravaged wife to die? Should a Missouri hospital refuse to withdraw life support from a comatose young woman named Nancy Cruzan even though her family believes there is no hope? Should a Minnesota hospital insist on withdrawing life support from a comatose older woman named Helga Wanglie despite the fact that her family believes there is still hope?

These questions seem dramatic and rare until you spend any time at all in a hospital. Then you realize that questions this complicated are asked every single day. Few reach the newspapers or become court cases, but each one causes pain and requires a solution, or something that pretends at a solution. Usually the best result is merely a half-hearted decision to accept one of two impossible choices.

And who answers these Solomonic questions? Hermann has formed a committee. It is called the Institutional Ethics Committee, and it meets whenever necessary in Room 3485. It has been doing so since 1983, and, back then, it was the only committee of its kind in the Texas Medical Center and one of the first in the nation. At that time, fewer than 4 percent of the country's hospitals had ethics committees. Within four years that number jumped to 60 percent, and eventually every major hospital in the United States will probably have one.

The topic the Hermann committee discusses most often is withdrawal of life support—whether and when to turn off the ventilator of a patient who cannot breathe on his own or remove a feeding tube from a patient who cannot feed himself. The topic the committee discusses least is money—whether the hospital can afford to provide a certain type of treatment.

A lovely myth, central to American society, pretends that money makes no difference. A hospital will not turn the poor from its doors, this fairy tale goes, and once a patient is inside, decisions about his care are based solely on medical need, rather than ability to pay. For life and death decisions, that is still primarily true. Laws and morals still require that lives be saved before insurance cards are checked. For all other decisions, however, money matters very much, a fact made clear by simply reading a patient's chart; the insurance status ("Blue Cross/Blue Shield," "Medicaid," "None") is stamped on every page. Ask Patrick's doctors who is paying the bill, and they will answer that Hermann probably will. If money were irrelevant, they would have no need to know.

Still, the committee has always agreed, without saying so directly, that costs are none of its concern. Its duty is to rise above any talk of dollars and cents or allocation of resources and carefully limit its conversations to what is ethical and just. But as the costs of medical care keep rising, discussions of money have been increasingly more difficult to avoid, at Hermann and in the rest of the medical world. So although money is rarely mentioned directly at meetings like this one, the unspoken subject is almost always there. Is Patrick a question of money? Is it unethical to think of the cost of his care or irresponsible not to? How much more should be done for a boy whose death is inevitable and who is costing the hospital hundreds of thousands of dollars a year?

There was a brief silence after Javier finished, and then Lin Weeks spoke up. A former intensive care nurse, she is now a vice-president of the hospital, in charge of the nurses in charge of many clinical services. It's an important job, and Lin is good at it, racing through her twelve-hour days, her date book as her guide, a marathon of conferencing, suggesting, brain-storming, and advising. She is also the chairman of the Ethics Committee. That job is her passion.

"Is there any remote possibility of curing him?" she asked Javier.

"No. He's a dying boy. We've all come to think he'll live forever, but Patrick is a dying kid."

"Are there any alternatives other than a new line?"

"I've looked into a full gut transplant, replacing everything. It has been done—in Russia, rarely, and I think there have been a few cases in Canada. But in both places all of them have died. Also, there's a surgeon at Baylor who's experimenting with stimulating the bowel to make it grow. It's promising, but Patrick's too sick for that."

With the mention of the transplant and the surgeons at another hospital, Richard Weir leaned forward, readying for a fight. Richard had known Patrick longer than almost anyone at Hermann, first as his play therapist and then as one of his closest friends.

"*That's* why I asked for this meeting, because people started talking about gut transplants and transfers," Richard said, gaining speed as he talked, stressing certain words for emphasis. "*Why* are we thinking of this?

Why are we thinking of sending this child, who is *so* dependent on his support system here, to another hospital, to surgeons at Baylor, to do something that has *no* chance of working?

"Even the simpler idea," he continued, "namely doing another surgery here to insert a new line. Why are we talking of putting him through that when we know it will make him miserable, it won't make him well, and it won't last?"

He shifted his gaze from Lin to Javier. "Are we doing this for *him* or are we doing this for *us*? Are we just too *attached* to him to let him go?"

One nurse standing in the back of the room broke rank with an answer: "You can't starve him to death. How can you give up?"

Hearing that, Kay Tittle shook her head and forgot her promise to keep quiet lest she get too emotional.

"There's a lot of hostility toward those of us, like Richard and me, who are talking about this," said Kay, Patrick's main nurse, a petite, solid woman, who blushes easily and is known throughout the hospital as Patrick's Other Mom.

She chose each word carefully—diplomacy is all in meetings like these—determined to make her point. "We're not giving up," she said. "*I'm* not giving up on him, but I can see what we're going to create. We talk a lot about quality of life, doing all of this to preserve his quality of life. Well, what would be quality of life for one child would not be a quality life for Patrick.

"What if we do this surgery, and he's still alive and we can't wean him off the ventilator?" she continued. "It's been getting harder every time. You know Patrick, it would destroy him to be that way. Why are we fighting so hard to keep him alive if he's going to be miserable?"

Javier's answer was almost a whisper, all but drowned out by the hum of the air-conditioning. He nodded, and his voice was sympathetic, but his words were not exactly what Kay wanted to hear.

"I also want him to have a quality life," he said. "I want to do anything he needs to enjoy life, and if that means doing another thoracotomy, opening his chest, so he can get around and do what he enjoys doing, so be it. Maybe that will make his life worse. But if we don't do it, he won't have a life."

He looked at Lin, then at Richard, then at Kay. "I need to know if this is the last line we can put in," he said. "I'm feeling very lonely with this decision."

Once again the room was silent. Over the past hour and a half all that needed saying had been said. Lin thanked everyone for coming and waited as the guests left and only the committee stayed seated. Javier didn't have to leave, since he was a committee member, but he knew he had no place at the decision-making part of this particular meeting. There was some shaking of hands and exchanges of social pleasantries as the visitors headed for the door, as if they were asking the committee to decide among a number of different business proposals rather than a number of different ways for a teenage boy to die.

A clipped, cold tone, distracting to an outsider, is standard at most meetings at hospitals. Just as police officers can drink coffee and tell jokes while standing next to a sheet-covered corpse, hospital staffers are matter-of-fact on the subject of death. Critics might use the word "hardened," and though that's accurate, it's also too simple. The emotional distance infuriates patients, but it keeps doctors sane. Most medical students are flattened by the first death of a patient, and that is as it should be. But if the doctor who has been practicing for twenty years still feels each death and downturn with the same intensity he felt the first time, he wouldn't be of much use to his patients.

So doctors look for a buffer zone, a barrier between themselves and what they do, a line that says, "I will give you this much of myself and no more." In hundreds of large and little ways the profession seeks to take something emotional, messy, unpredictable, and unstructured, and tries to give it form. When the patient does X, the doctor does Y. When it's 10 A.M., it's time for rounds. When faced with an ethical dilemma, take it to a committee. Make it neat and ordered, part of an agenda.

Once the visitors had left, the entire Hermann Hospital Ethics Committee proceeded to disagree politely. The conversation turned staccato, bouncing around the table from member to member.

"Would it help to ask Patrick what he wants?"

"He's fifteen years old, he's just a kid."

"It's his life."

"They would have to ask him if we made him DNR."

"Are we suggesting that? No one asked us about Do Not Resuscitate."

"I think we should suggest that. In a way that's what they *were* asking. 'How much more do we do?' Not resuscitating is an answer to that question."

"Will his mother agree?"

"Last time she said, 'Whatever the doctor says.' This time she didn't want to come. She told Javier, 'Whatever the doctors says.' "

"Would DNR mean no surgery?"

"I would think so. It's a decision to hold back. Another surgery is hardly holding back."

"There's no right answer to this one."

"Is there ever?"

Halfway through the conversation Randy Gleason, the hospital's lawyer, began to scribble on the yellow and white form titled "Advisory Opinion of the Institutional Ethics Committee." In the space labeled "Specific Issue to Be Considered," he wrote, "Considering the patient's terminal prognosis and current quality of life, should extraordinary medical measures be initiated or continued?" In answer, he wrote: "The opinion of the Institutional Ethics Committee is that it would be appropriate to initiate Supportive Protocol II," the hospital policy that allows doctors to stop fighting to cure patients or even keep them alive, requiring only that they be kept "comfortable." After everyone signed the form, Randy checked the box labeled "unanimous."

Javier was waiting on a stiff-backed foam-filled couch outside Room 3485 when Lin walked out and gave him a copy of the form. He carried it down the hall, where Patrick was sleeping, and slipped it into the boy's chart. But that was hardly the end of the story. One rule of medicine is that illness doesn't read the textbooks. This would not be the last meeting, official or otherwise, about Patrick.

JUNE

Taylor and Jake

In a drab room in the high-risk obstetrics unit, Fran Poarch was about to lose both her babies. Lying on the narrow stainless steel bed, she squeezed her eyes shut to make the fear go away, then opened them again to watch the two $25,000 fetal monitors that blipped and beeped by her side. She was certain that if she kept her eyes closed for too long, the peaks and valleys on the screen would dissolve into ominous straight lines.

The monitors showed the babies' hearts were beating 140 times a minute, normal, but alarming to watch when Fran compared them to the slower designs etched on another monitor by her own racing heart. A fourth screen showed she was having contractions every three or four minutes. They weren't strong enough for her to feel, and she only knew they were happening when the monitor began to jump.

So it was fear, not pain, that kept her fingers dug into the thick, narrow mattress. Even the drugs she had been given to make her muscles relax weren't powerful enough to stop the clenching. The medications were to fight her contractions and keep the twins from being born. The babies weren't due for four more months, but already her cervix was dilated one-third as far as it could go, and their arrival impossible to prevent. She tried not to breathe too deeply, as if the very act of breathing would fill her up with air and push the babies out.

In the moments when she dared to look around, Fran was surprised by the dreariness of the hospital, and she wondered if she had been taken to the wrong place by mistake. Her confusion grew when a doctor strode in with a stack of Houston telephone books nearly too high to carry. Without explanation, the woman lifted up the foot of Fran's bed and shoved the books underneath the steel legs. The plan was to keep her on a slant, with her head more than 3 feet lower than her toes, so the babies wouldn't press against her cervix. Her world was now officially upside down.

A week earlier her world had been close to perfect. Married to her best friend from high school, living comfortably in a picture book home in the country club outskirts of Houston, she was having an easy pregnancy and her biggest worry was whether to use a duck or bunny motif in the nursery. Then, on the last day in May, she went for her regular monthly checkup. She had expected a one-hour interruption of her day, but the visit soon became much more serious than that. "Your cervix is thinned out a little," Dr. Jane Reed explained, and sent Fran home with a prescription for terbutaline, a drug that can help stop premature labor. She was not to get out of bed for four days, and then she was to come in and be looked at again.

It was raining that Friday morning, and Fran wanted to skip the follow-up appointment. She was sure the drugs had worked. After all, she felt lazy from bed rest but otherwise healthy. Carey, her husband of less than a year, wouldn't allow her to stay home, and he wouldn't allow her to drive herself either. They kept the appointment and learned that the drugs had definitely not worked. Fran's cervix was nearly 4 centimeters dilated

(10 centimeters is the last stage of labor) and 90 percent effaced, or thinned.

From there everything moved quickly. Dr. Reed eased Fran onto a stretcher, ignoring her protests that she needed to stand up and put her pants back on. In the interest of modesty her legs were covered with a sheet as Dr. Reed wheeled her through the waiting room, out of the medical office building, and into the Woodlands Community Hospital, which was next door. "Don't sit up, Fran," the anxious doctor said during the bumpy trip. "I'm very serious, Fran. This is very serious."

Her doctors had called Hermann's LifeFlight helicopter-ambulance, which landed in their parking lot twenty minutes later. Fran hated the idea of a helicopter and asked why she couldn't go by car.

"I'll lay down and stay still," she promised, afraid that, by accepting the chopper, she would also have to accept what was happening to her.

"Driving will be too dangerous in the rain," the emergency room doctor said.

"Oh, yeah, I love the thought of a *helicopter* in the rain."

The trip, made bumpier by the weather, took twenty minutes, and as soon as Fran was wheeled through the back door of Hermann, she wanted to leave.

Massive and intense, Hermann Hospital is very different from the small, almost friendly community hospital that she had just left. Hermann actually has three "front doors," each belonging to an addition that was built to be the final word in medical care in Houston, at least until the next one came along. The original front door, built in 1925, looks like the entrance to anything but a hospital—two dark oak panels under a limestone archway engraved with winged lions and clinging vines. The entrance to this building, named after two benefac-

tors, Hugh Roy and Lillie Cranz Cullen, leads to a cob-
blestoned courtyard, with more relief sculpture and a
gurgling fountain in the middle.

Hermann's second front door was added only twenty
years later, in 1945, because the visionaries of the post-
war boom viewed the original charm as obsolete. The
old building was adequate for the charity patients (and
the black patients), according to the thinking at the
time. But paying patients deserved a state-of-the-art
building, one that reflected a new world of medicine
and was shiny, efficient, and unsentimental. The front
door of *this* building, called the Corbin J. and
Wilhelmina C. Robertson Pavilion, would never be of
wood, but of two banks of aluminum and glass on a flat
brick facade. No cluttered Moorish drama here, just
aqua tiled walls, gray linoleum floors, and cramped,
echoing rooms that feel dark no matter what the wattage
of the fluorescent tubes.

In 1972, the hospital's newest entrance was added, in
the form of the Jesse H. and Mary Gibbs Jones Pavilion. These doors open automatically as patients approach, sliding into walls of sand-colored concrete.
Brighter than the second building and blander than the
first, this section of Hermann is sterile in its efficiency.

The helipad is atop a parking garage outside Robertson, the wartime vintage entrance, and the hallways of
institutional green tile are the first thing that conscious
LifeFlight patients see. It seemed to Fran that dozens of
people converged on her helicopter when it landed. Actually there were only about eight, most from Obstetrics
and Pediatrics, which had been alerted that she had arrived. Some of the people pushed her stretcher while
others followed only steps behind pushing the monitors,
which were still attached to her arms and abdomen. The

entire parade raced into the elevator and to the high-risk maternity unit on the dark third floor of Robertson.

It was there, lying on an awkward slant, that Fran first met Dr. Sharon Crandell, who was in charge of the preemie nursery during the month of June. Sharon chose her words carefully and spoke in a flat, business-like tone, an approach she believes is the best way to get through to emotion-shocked people.

Twenty-five weeks is not nearly enough time for the babies to become fully developed, Sharon explained, which is why a full-term pregnancy is at least thirty-eight weeks. Not that a baby born in this era of medicine needs all thirty-eight weeks in order to survive. But the longer the twins stayed put, the better their chances.

Sharon's specialty, neonatology, is an aggressive, in-trusive, no-holds-barred branch of medicine, and it tends to attract doctors who fit that description. They don't go into this subspecialty to give up or to have doubts. Their purpose is to keep a patch of flesh alive long enough for it to become a baby.

They are winning that fight, and the age at which a preemie can be saved has crept steadily lower, with progress quite literally being measured in days. Not too long ago doctors automatically gave up on thirty-weekers. A year before Fran landed at Hermann, it was considered rare to save a twenty-seven-weeker. Now the line was thought to be at twenty-five or twenty-six weeks and moving lower.

There are a lot of reasons for these changes, and Sharon explained some of them to Fran. She began with the mysteries of surfactant, a thick, white, oily sub-stance, that smells somewhat like fish, and coats the tiny air sacs of the lung. The job of surfactant is to keep those sacs open slightly after the lungs are emptied, in anticipation of the next breath. Without it, the sacs would collapse flat and be more difficult to inflate—the difference between blowing up a balloon that's completely compressed and one that still has a little air. The lungs often don't start to produce surfactant until the thirty-third week of pregnancy. Without it, the baby can exhaust himself simply by trying to breathe.

There is a way to speed up the process and produce surfactant before the thirty-third week. As with so many other medical discoveries, this one came about by accident. In 1972, a researcher in New Zealand, who had been looking for something completely different, found that when he injected certain steroids into pregnant sheep, their premature lambs were born with fully developed lungs. He tried doing the same to human subjects—women in premature labor—and showed that, if labor could be slowed long enough for a twenty-four-to-forty-eight-hour course of steroids to be given, the premature babies were likely to have healthier lungs.

That, Sharon said, was why Fran was lying on an uncomfortable slant. Without expounding on the sheep in New Zealand, Sharon described the danger of lung disease in preemies.

"The fetuses would very likely not be viable at this point," she said. "They need time. The obstetricians want to keep giving you drugs to stop your labor and then give you the steroids to help their lungs."

"Will that work?" asked Fran's mother, who had driven to Hermann with Carey.

"Let's hope so," Sharon said, and left the room.

Neither hope nor terbutaline was enough. Fran spent the night on an angle, sleeping fitfully, waking up in sync with the contractions, which were coming every fifteen minutes or so. Her mother slept equally poorly in the chair next to her bed, covered with a thin hospital blanket. Carey didn't sleep at all. He lay on the floor, a pillow propped beneath his head, and watched the monitors that the nurses had taught him to read.

By morning it was obvious that the labor was not going to stop. Fran's cervix was dilated to 7 centimeters and Dr. Patty Ross, a high-risk obstetrician, told them, "There's not much more we can do." As she spoke, two nurses came in and removed the telephone books that were wedged under the legs of the bed, kicking them into a corner like the unscientific last-ditch effort that they were.

Dr. Ross asked Fran and Carey what they wanted done for the babies, if the expected didn't happen, and they were born alive.

"Do everything," Carey said, and Fran nodded her agreement. "Do everything possible to save my kids. Do more than what's possible."

The labor progressed slowly. Fran's cervix refused to stay closed, but it also refused to dilate completely and drugs were used to help the process along. Although the telephone books were removed at dawn, Fran wasn't wheeled into the delivery room until 2:40 that afternoon. It was a surreal form of emotional torture: wishing something would never happen and at the same time hoping it would happen faster. Carey paced the tiny room, feeling like an imposter in his green surgical scrubs. Fran thought about the Lamaze classes she hadn't taken and hoped she would know what to do when the babies started to come.

She still couldn't feel the contractions, and her eyes rarely left the monitor that told her what her body was doing. Finally, when the fluorescent peaks were as high as they were likely to go, she was wheeled into the delivery room, four doors down the hall, Room 412. As her bed passed through the doorway she squeezed the hand closest to her and whispered, "I'm scared." The nurse squeezed back.

The room was crowded, with two obstetricians for Fran and a full team of pediatricians for each twin. Dr. Ross was at the foot of the table, ready to deliver the babies. Sharon Crandell stood in back of her, against the wall, waiting to take over as soon as the first child was born. Even before the umbilical cords were cut, this would cease being an obstetrical problem and begin being her problem. Two nurses stood at Fran's shoulders, giving her a crash course in how to have a baby: "You're doing great, hon, really great. Now push real hard, just like on television."

Carey felt cold. The tiled walls and floors, the stainless steel and the mirrors, the masked faces that made it impossible to tell whom he had already met and who at this intimate gathering were strangers, they all gave the room an added chill.

When the first baby was born at 3:18, Dr. Ross looked up at him and shook her head. "She's small, Carey," she said. "It's going to be tough."

Carey felt even colder.

Lee Taylor Poarch, 1 pound, 8 ounces, gave a short, delayed cry before Sharon's practiced hands suctioned the fluid out of her lungs, slid a tube down her throat, and attached her to a machine to help her breathe. Fran couldn't see Taylor and was surprised to hear her cry at all. She thought to herself, "I guess this means she isn't dead."

Carey was able to hold the baby for a moment after the tubes were in and before she was whisked off to the intensive care nursery. With no body fat to protect her, Taylor was bruised from head to toe during birth. She had ten fingers and ten toes—Carey felt silly, but counted anyway. The tiny girl fit in the palm of her father's hand, with her head at Carey's wrist and her feet hanging slightly over his middle finger.

Jacob Carey Poarch arrived at 4:44, an hour and a half later. He was a little bigger than his sister, weighing 1 pound and 15 ounces, but his birth was more complicated. The umbilical cord was wrapped twice around his neck. Jake cried too, weakly but definitely, until the same tubes silenced him in order to save his life.

Fran was exhausted. Not from the delivery itself, which she had barely felt at all, but from emotion, drugs, and lack of sleep. For the past twenty-four hours, she had been lying all but on her head with nothing to eat but chips of ice. She fell into a deep sleep in the recovery room at five o'clock and didn't wake up for two hours. Carey was there when she opened her eyes. He had signed the babies' birth certificates, and he had been to the nursery for a few minutes to see them. But he and Fran didn't talk about that. There was too much to say and no easy place to begin.

So they talked about the overnight bag Carey had packed after Fran left in the helicopter and the fact that he remembered his own toothbrush and pajamas, but had forgotten to bring anything for Fran to wear. Carey's mother went to the store across the street and returned with a bathrobe and slippers. An orderly came with a wheelchair and brought the young, frightened couple to a room on the regular medical floor—away from other women who were having babies. Another excuse for more blessed small talk. Using a checklist, the nurse upstairs showed them where the telephone was, how the call light worked, and how to move the mechanical bed into a more comfortable position.

Eventually there was nothing left to do but go see Jake and Taylor. Fran was afraid. Imagination can be worse than reality, and hers had been working full throttle for several hours. Carey wheeled her chair to the neonatal intensive care unit, taught her how to scrub to the elbows at the giant steel sinks, then guided her to the side-by-side warmers that held her twins. They lay on platforms on rolling carts, each with a heat lamp above them and a fluffy white pad, a man-made sheepskin rug, as a mattress.

They were tinier than Fran had imagined, but sweeter and more helpless, too. She had expected the thicket of tubes and wires that regulated and measured every body function. What she hadn't expected was that they would look so much like babies, miniature, translucent babies, and her heart ached watching the effort they were making simply to breathe. Even from a distance she could see their ribs flutter in and out, in and out, with each hiccup of a breath.

Unable to hold their children, Fran and Carey asked questions. Dr. Joe Mendiola, who was on call in the nursery that night, answered patiently.

What's the purpose of each tube?

The blue plastic tubes in their mouths are the ventilator, attached to a computer that regulates the speed at which they breathe and the percentage of pure oxygen in each of those breaths. The round patch stuck to their chest is to measure their heartbeat. The one next to it measures their respiration rate. The needles in their arms bring medication and nutrition. The thin wires protruding from where their belly buttons will be are threaded into an umbilical artery and vein, making it easy to get blood samples whenever they're needed, which can be often, and to give IV fluids. The patches over their eyes are to protect them from the bright fluorescent lights right over the crib, which in turn prevent jaundice.

Do the IVs hurt?

They pinch for a moment when the needle pierces the skin, but they don't really hurt after that.

Can they hear what's going on?

When they're awake. They sleep very deeply.

When will they be able to see?

When the eye patches come off. They won't see well, no newborn does, but they will probably be able to see.

How are they doing?

We wish they were doing better. Taylor seems stronger than Jake, even though Jake is a little bit bigger. Girls born prematurely seem to do better as a rule than do premature boys. We don't know why, we just know that it's true.

Will Taylor live through the night?

We think so.

Will Jake?

We're not sure.

Though the doctor was kind, Fran and Carey felt awkward, like they were getting in the way. They said their good-byes, first to Jake and then to Taylor, and went back to Fran's room. Suddenly ravenous, they ordered a pizza.

About an hour later Dr. Mendiola called. Taylor's condition was unchanged, he said, but Jake's breathing was steadily worse. Would they like to have him christened?

By the time they arrived back upstairs, the chaplain was waiting for them by their son's isolette. The ceremony was short and cold, another bedside hospital procedure. Carey held Jake while the priest dabbed water on the baby's forehead. Fran was afraid to hold her son, certain that he would break in her hand. She left as quickly as she could, but Carey stayed behind and talked to Jake, stroking the baby's back ever so lightly in rhythm with his words.

"I love you very much," he said. "You'll always be my first boy. You'll always be with me, wherever I go.

"Don't be afraid," he said. "You're going to the biggest playground in the world. One day I'll see you there. I'll see you there real soon."

He pulled a Kleenex from a nearby flowered box, but he didn't dab his eyes until he left the room.

Carey and Fran tried to sleep, but succeeded only in lying in the dark, eyes closed and jaws tense, waiting for a tap at the door. It came two hours later, a stranger's voice telling them that Jake had died a few minutes earlier, at 1:07 A.M.

Fran and Carey called their parents, then cried most of the night in a wet, convulsing embrace. At some point they fell asleep, knocked out by all the tears, only to awake hours later and ache all over again.

In the morning, as early as Fran's doctor would allow it, they made a quick visit to Taylor, trying to look everywhere but the spot that had held Jake's bed. Then they fled Hermann, past the smiling new mothers who left carrying babies and flowers and a belief that the world was fair. They drove home in relative silence, picked at the huge breakfast their families had busied themselves preparing, slept for several hours, then drove back to Hermann to visit Taylor.

Soon they would know every inch of that drive by heart.

Patrick

Two days after the stormy meeting of the Ethics Committee, a smaller, even more emotional meeting was held in the tiny conference room on the pediatrics floor. Everyone who attended called it a "family meeting" about Patrick, despite the fact that only one of the five people at the round Formica table was actually related to the boy, and she got there late.

Richard Weir was the first to arrive. He took a seat facing the door, with his back to the small window. Alone for a few moments, he doodled squares and circles on the table top with his finger. Sally Olsen, Javier's assistant, arrived next. She headed directly for the telephone on the wall and answered a page she had received while she was walking from her office. While Sally was dialing, Kay Tittle came in. She walked quickly, afraid she was late, but slowed her pace when she saw the room was still relatively empty. She took a chair next to Richard. Sally ended her call and sat across from them both. The three made uncomfortable small talk, checking the wall clock constantly and wondering whether Javier Aceves and Patrick's mother would arrive before they ran out of things to say.

When twenty minutes passed and the number of people in the room had not changed, Sally decided to

begin the meeting herself. There was no knowing
when Javier would appear, she reasoned, since he was
chronically late, the result of his policy never to cut
short a conversation with a patient, or a parent, or
anyone else for that matter. And she was fairly certain
that Oria Dismuke would not arrive at all. Patrick's
mother often avoided meetings at which she thought
the news might be bad.

So Sally started this meeting the way nearly every
meeting in the hospital begins, with a brief history of
the case. "I've seen Javier do it a thousand times so
I guess I can, too," she said self-consciously before
she began. Neither Kay nor Richard broke a smile.

The tension was typical of meetings about Patrick.
It was an uneasiness that had only a little to do with
the life and death issues being discussed and everything to do with Patrick himself. At age fifteen he
was the size of an eight-year-old and practically the
hospital mascot. When he walked through the halls,
everyone—doctors, dietary staff, security guards—all
said hello. If asked, more Hermann employees could
probably recognize Patrick than the hospital's CEO.

That's because the CEO is not fond of popping
wheelies in the hallways in a wheelchair. Patrick is.
He can also be found selling his crayoned drawings
for 25 cents each in the lobby. One night, a security
guard received an anonymous call from a patient saying there was a dead body under a bed. Unflustered,
the guard called the pediatric nurses' station and told
them that Patrick was playing pranks with the telephone again.

Although everyone knows Patrick, some know him
better than others, and those invited to this meeting
were the ones who know him best. He has been in
Richard's life the longest, ten years, since the boy was

five years old and Richard was a newcomer to his job. That job is playing with children as a form of therapy, and Richard looks the part, with his shaggy beard and zany suspenders, the kind that are likely to be decorated with waddling penguins.

Patrick casts rapid spells, and it didn't take long before Richard became his best friend. He was drawn to the boy's cocky attitude and the vulnerability hidden underneath. Once, when Patrick was ten but looked like six, Richard took him to a sporting goods show at the cavernous Houston Astrodome. The boy ran around wide eyed for hours looking at the equipment for countless sports he was simply too frail to play. Near the end of the afternoon, in a corner booth at the show, Patrick spotted a vintage jacket from a Houston Cougars basketball team. The white leather coat had flaming red letters sewn in an arc on the back. When he tried it on, its sleeves touched the floor and its waist reached his ankles. But he pronounced it a "radical looking coat," and Richard bought it for him. He wore it all day and for years after that, and every time he did his body language changed. His shoulders shot up and back until it seemed that they might meet, and his strides became loping and long. It was as if he decided he was tall. Richard loved that about him.

Richard is drawn to Patrick's independence. Kay Tittle is drawn to Patrick's neediness. She met Patrick when he was ten years old, the year she began work as a nurse at Hermann. At first he kept his distance, asking the more familiar nurses about her but not paying her direct attention. Then one day, without warning, his primary nurse, who had been at Hermann almost since he was born, resigned to take another job. She called Kay aside and said, "I'm giving you Patrick. He and I discussed it, and he decided he wanted you." Kay's husband, Denzial, still teases her about that afternoon, when she came home and announced, "They gave Patrick to me today."

"What do you mean they *gave* you Patrick."

"Patrick's mine."

Ownership of the child meant that within months he had become a part of her family. Kay and Denzial would take him on field trips—to the airport to watch the planes take off was a favorite. They would take him to dinner, though dinner for him was not like dinner for most children, since he couldn't eat any real food. He would go to McDonald's to nibble on an apple pie and take a few sips of a Sprite. It was the *idea* of going out to dinner that appealed to him.

Before every surgery, he would call Kay, usually between midnight and 6 A.M. He knew she would be asleep, but he took comfort in the fact that she loved him enough to wake herself up to talk. The conversations were full of silence:

"Hi."

"Hi."

"What are you doing?"

"I was sleeping."

Then they would each breathe into the phone for a while until Patrick would finally say, "Well, I'd better get back to sleep." Kay would respond, "I'll see you in the morning." They both understood this was their way of saying, "I'm scared," and, "I know you are, but I'll be there for you."

The fierce attachment Kay and Richard feel for Patrick is a burden to Javier Aceves, who knows he is responsible for one of the most beloved children at Hermann. By the time the Ethics Committee met to talk about Patrick in May, Javier had been the boy's primary physician for only eight months, but he had known him much longer than that, since the days when Javier was a medical resident at Hermann. Theirs is a complicated relationship, a reflection of two complicated people.

Javier has always been drawn to issues of life, death, and children. Growing up in Mexico, he had planned to study theology and become a Jesuit priest, but after several summers working at missions in dusty rural villages, teaching families about health and sanitation, he decided that he needed to have a family of his own. Barely twenty years old, he married Roseanne, whom he had known since childhood, and entered medical school in Mexico City. He planned to be a country doctor, caring for Indian mountain villages, but that, he says, was "B.C.," Before Children. They had three sons by his last year of medical school (over the years there would be a daughter, too), and he changed his plans again, deciding to open a pediatrics practice closer to Mexico City, where there were good schools and hospitals for his family.

He was weeks away from beginning his pediatrics residency when two-year-old Francisco, one of a set of twins, was diagnosed with cancer. Afraid to trust the system that had trained him, Javier brought the boy, known as Paco, to Houston's M. D. Anderson Cancer Center for a second opinion. The verdict there was consistent with what the doctors in Mexico had said: His baby would need chemotherapy; there was no guarantee he would survive the treatment; if he did survive the short term, it would be years before he could be declared cured.

Javier returned to Mexico for several days, sold the few pieces of furniture he owned, then moved back to Houston with his family, expecting to stay for about two years. His medical training was on indefinite hold, and he had no idea what work he would find to pay for groceries once in Texas. He was prepared to wait tables or labor in a factory if necessary.

The doctors who cared for Paco stepped in and offered more than medical hope. They also offered Javier a future, in the form of a job at Anderson, as a resident in their pediatrics program. The pay was better than he would have earned in Mexico, even accounting for the difference in the cost of living. And there was an obvious advantage. On those days that Paco spent in the hospital, with an IV line dripping cancer-killing chemicals into his arm, Javier could duck out from work to say hello to his son.

The three-year residency made Javier all the more sensitive to the suffering of children, and the anger he felt surprised him. In Mexico he had been frustrated at what medicine was unable to do. In Houston, at one of the most sophisticated medical centers in the world, he was increasingly frustrated at what medicine was able to do. He came home from long nights and spilled his confusion to Roseanne in slow, almost whispered monologues.

"Medical centers are good at acute care, at saving people, but they aren't as good at the chronic care, the aftermath of being saved," he would say. "Congenital heart defects, severe infections, severe traumas, near drownings, everyone has a good chance. We can make them okay, but we can't always make them the same as before, or the same as other kids. So then these families go home and have to live with what we did, and we don't always give them enough help after that. Shouldn't the responsibility go further than patching them up and sending them away?"

The monologues were deepest and most anguished

during his first Christmas in Houston. Many people look back on their lives and wonder how they got where they are. Javier knows that his life changed radically that Christmas Eve, when a two-year-old girl named Latasha was brought into the emergency room, then up to the ICU, where he was working. She was a wrenching sight, with burns over 90 percent of her body, everywhere but on her scalp and the soles of her feet. For two months Javier worked to keep the girl alive, ordering excruciating baths every day, during which the dead charred skin was scraped away so new scarred skin might grow. As the weeks passed, he found himself looking at her face, which he knew would be marginally functional, but never presentable, even after years of plastic surgery. He imagined her as a teenager, when her peers were beginning to date. He knew she would be angry.

"She'll want to know, 'Why did you save me?' " he whispered to Roseanne. "And I won't be there to answer. I don't have an answer, but I owe her one. I owe her more than just saving her and sending her off into the world without ever helping her again."

Latasha died eight weeks after Christmas, and Javier was relieved. It was three more years before he could act on the decision he made during the months he cared for her, but when he finished his residency, he opened a clinic at Hermann for the children, like Latasha, who belong to no one. His patients are the chronically ill, with conditions that will debilitate them throughout their lifetimes and eventually kill them. These are the patients whom other doctors cannot or will not handle. The average pediatrician sees only a handful of children like this during years of practice and is not accustomed to answering their needs. In fact, many would prefer not to care for them at all. There are glib generalizations about every specialty in medicine—surgery is aggressive and arrogant, dermatology has easy schedules, cardiology is a gold mine. The common description of pediatrics is that it provides less money than some other specialties, but a lot more hope. Most children get sick and then get better. That means pediatrics is one of the few specialties where good news is the norm. But Javier's patients will never get better, and that emotional drain is more than many pediatricians are prepared to accept.

Which is why 130 children depend on Javier. Technically, he is a medical school employee, earning a straight salary and using the school's office space and the hospital's medical facilities. In practice, however, he runs an independent clinic that simply happens to be located in a hospital building. He calls his creation CHOSEN, and his patients are "the chosen ones." The acronym is fudged a bit because he liked the word and was determined to find something for it to stand for. So the full name of the clinic is Chronic Health Oriented Services for Niños.

His patients have every imaginable problem: cerebral palsy, autism, mental retardation, spina bifida, head trauma from car accidents, and gunshot wounds. The only thing they have in common is that their particular illness or injury defines nearly every part of their lives. So CHOSEN is designed to do more than provide regular checkups and occasional emergency visits. It has a data bank of physical therapists, speech therapists, and special education teachers. It can plug patients into church groups or charitable organizations that might help when the bills get too high. It has been known to speed up the delivery of a custom-made wheelchair, discreetly locate the nearest food bank, or arrange for a hospital van to drive a patient to an appointment when the family car refuses to cooperate.

CHOSEN has a monthly newsletter, a parent support group, and a phone number parents can call at any time of day or night. House calls are routine, although Javier prefers to call them "home visits."

"It's hard to bring a kid in on a ventilator," he says. "You can hire an ambulance, but it's easier for me to go myself."

His patients and their parents adore him, and there are a lot of hugs dispensed along with the prescriptions. He knows what these parents are feeling. Even though his son Paco is in remission, Javier knows the fear, the frustration, and the anger that descend when a child is terribly sick. Sometimes he tells the parents his son's story, but only when he thinks it will help. Every family needs something different, he has learned, and whereas some might take strength from his happy ending, others would feel only anger that such an ending wasn't possible for them.

There are many who think Javier can walk on water, but even he cannot run a clinic this emotionally draining and administratively complicated alone. Sally Olsen is the other half of CHOSEN, the combination nurse, social worker, counselor, secretary, and office manager. She is a soft, friendly woman, with a sharp Texas twang, a sharp tongue, and an even sharper sense of herself. Like Javier, she is on a mission. She had a daughter who died at birth twenty-five years ago, and her marriage broke up during the months afterward, when she needed to talk about the baby and her husband needed to forget.

"No one talked about death then," she said. "They

were scared shitless. Still are. Death and I are old friends. There's no shame in it."

Depending on the observer, Sally is either an oddball or a saint. In the carefully scripted world of medicine, she regularly says things that are designed to get attention, and she succeeds. For instance, she believes she is psychically connected to people, especially patients. Every so often a CHOSEN patient will die, and Sally will sense his or her death. More than once, she says, she has sat upright in bed, looked at her clock, and simply known that something had happened. She describes the clanging sound she heard early one particular morning, like that of a big metal door slamming shut, and she was certain she had heard the gates of heaven closing behind a patient she particularly loved. Within an hour, there was a phone call from the hospital telling her that patient had died.

Javier thinks this is strange, but he doesn't dwell on it. He knows that CHOSEN would not run without Sally. She is the one who, more often than not, speeds the delivery of wheelchairs, finds the food banks, and prods Javier to get to meetings on time. Her ability to finesse the Hermann Hospital bureaucracy annoys many who are not as good at blustering and cajoling, but it earns her Javier's gratitude.

One place she has not talked her way into, however, is the tight circle around Patrick. Although CHOSEN is at the center of the boy's day-to-day medical care, Sally and Javier are very much the outsiders when it comes to the rest of his life. When he is in pain, he calls Javier, but when he needs a hug, he calls Richard, Kay, or a handful of other nonmedical staff.

That bothers Javier more than it bothers Sally, which is surprising since she is treated with open annoyance while he is respected, although from a distance. Sally is often excluded from meetings about Patrick's care or snapped at when she does attend. No one would think of excluding Javier, although the repartee at the conference table sounds forced when he is around.

Sally reacts by making a virtue of the cold shoulders. "If they have to be mad at somebody, and they can't be mad at God, it might as well be me, 'cause I can sure handle it," she tells her second husband, Ken, a sympathetic minister.

Javier reacts by heaping extra pressure on himself. Over the months, Patrick has become more than just another one of 130 patients to Javier. He has become a test of the concept on which CHOSEN is based, that a chronically ill patient needs a mentor to help him through the medical maze. Javier trained under the senior doctors at Hermann, and now, supposedly, he was their colleague. But it takes more than a title change to make an underling suddenly feel like an equal. It also takes action. And the way Javier sees it, his first dramatic action might be to let the hospital's favorite patient die.

"I've just come into this, and he's going to die with me being his doctor," he said to Sally late one afternoon in early summer, when Patrick was still in the ICU and a booming thunderstorm outside made everything seem even more dramatic.

"Javier, you're not killing him," Sally answered. "His body is telling us it's time."

Sally was nearly ten minutes into her summary to an unsmiling Richard and Kay when Javier finally walked in.

"I was just giving a history," Sally said.

"We all know his history," Javier said matter-of-factly, not intending to embarrass Sally, but doing so quite effectively.

Javier took a seat, opened a notebook, uncapped a pen, and placed it gently on the table. Then he leaned back in his chair and looked toward Richard. "I think the Ethics Committee was helpful," he said. "It helped clarify the choices, and it made me feel less alone with this decision. The committee was a good idea."

His thank-you remained unspoken but understood.

"Well, what's our plan?" Sally asked.

"I think we should make him DNR," Javier said.

Everyone nodded. They all understood the hospital shorthand for Do Not Resuscitate, and they also understood the significance for Patrick. The term DNR is most commonly used in its literal sense—if a patient's heart stops beating or he stops breathing, he will not be saved, or, in hospital language, he will not be "coded." No one will pound on his chest, zap him with electricity, or inject him with drugs designed to make his heart restart. No one will fill his lungs with air so that his brain is not deprived of oxygen. He will be allowed to die.

DNR is relatively new. Orders *not* to resuscitate are an outgrowth of the ability *to* resuscitate, and cardiopulmonary resuscitation wasn't fully developed until after 1960. The so-called crash carts, with all the equipment needed to resuscitate a patient, were not used at Hermann until 1965. In those earliest days, there was nothing official about making a patient DNR. It was something doctors would do almost in secret, often without consulting the patient or the family. The staff would decide among themselves that a patient would be better off if he weren't resuscitated, and by general agreement he would not be. Sometimes, for the sake of appearances, rather than perform a "no code" the staff might perform a "slow code," going through the motions but without the speed or urgency needed for success.

The 1970s and 1980s brought two contradictory reactions to the hush-hush approach to DNR. First, the consumer rights movement led patients to demand control over health care in general and end-of-life decisions in particular. Patients wanted DNR, but they wanted it out in the open, and they wanted to make the decision themselves. At the same time, the case of Karen Ann Quinlan in 1976, in which a court ordered the creation of a committee to review the decision of doctors on whether life-support should be removed, made many doctors feel that someone was literally looking over their shoulder. That, coupled with a dramatic rise in malpractice suits, made doctors hesitant about writing any order that could create any sort of legal trouble. In particular, they balked at writing an order to allow a patient to die. DNR came to a de facto halt. In reaction to the confusion, hospitals hunkered down and formed committees.

One of the first decisions the Hermann Ethics Committee made was about DNR. What they actually decided was to stop calling it DNR, a step that was not quite as esoteric as it sounds. Their basic assumption was that DNR is a good thing, allowing patients to die with some dignity and curtailing futile medical care. Yet they found that many doctors and families were hesitant to ask that a patient be made DNR. After hours of discussion and unscientific polling of colleagues over lunch and in hallways, they decided that the term itself was having a chilling effect. Few other orders in medicine are phrased in such absolute negatives. Everything else is active: Give the following drugs at the following times, conduct the following tests, monitor the following symptoms. The words *Do Not* made doctors feel that they were shirking their responsibilities and made families feel that they were abandoning their loved ones.

So DNR orders at Hermann are officially known as Supportive Care Protocols. The committee felt that the new official term summed up what DNR is all about—keeping patients comfortable until they die—but did so in more positive terms. It evoked active images of caring and comforting rather than passive images of standing aside and watching a patient die.

There are two types of Supportive Protocols at Hermann. Category I covers what is traditionally meant by DNR: Everything will be done to keep the patient alive until the point at which his heartbeat or breathing stops. Then nothing will be done. Category II is more complicated. It allows doctors to withdraw other types of treatment in addition to last-ditch resuscitation. Under Supportive Protocol II, dialysis on a terminal kidney patient may be stopped if it is thought to be causing more agony than relief. Antibiotics may be withdrawn, a ventilator may be removed, and surgery may be forgone. The policy, as set in writing by the committee, allows a menu of procedures that may be stopped if they are determined to be futile in curing the patient and are simply postponing death.

Despite the shiny new terminology, most of the staff still uses the letters DNR. So everyone understood what Javier meant when he said that he wanted to issue a DNR order for Patrick. And despite the fact that under the mix-and-match policy, this could mean the withdrawal of a variety of things, they knew what Javier had in mind. He wasn't planning on removing the boy from the ventilator or stopping his antibiotics, because those were still making him more comfortable than he would

be if they weren't there. But he was saying, more finally than he ever had before, that there would be no
more surgery. And he was also saying that, if Patrick
actively started to die, the staff would stand back and
allow him to do so, giving painkillers to make his death
easier but not actively intervening to keep his body
working.

As Richard heard the words, he gave an involuntary
sigh. He realized that this was what he had been waiting
to hear for more than a year.

"I think that makes sense," he said. "I know that's
easy for me to say because I'm not the one who has
to write the order, but I think it's the right thing."

"Patrick is a dying child," Javier said, and everyone
in the room knew how hard it was for him to speak that
simple sentence. "We treat him like he'll beat the odds
because he always does, but it's time we face the fact
that he is a dying boy."

"Does he know that?" Sally asked.

Richard swayed his head slightly from side to side,
a move that was a cross between a nod "yes" and a
shake "no" and which was meant to indicate precisely
that.

"It's not like he hasn't thought about death," he said,
his mind forming a picture of a few other children, who,
like Patrick, relied on liquid food called "total paren-
teral nutrition," or TPN.

"It used to be him, Christie, José, and Jason, here on
the floor all the time for their TPN," he said. "Since
none of them could eat, they became real tight with
each other. Then Christie died right about the time that
José died, and Patrick went and said good-bye to them
both.

"He and Jason tried to make it into a joke," Richard

continued. "They'd say, 'Well, Christie's down. Well, José's dead. Which of us is going to be next?' "

Sally interrupted. "But did you ever really talk to them about it?"

"That was about as much as he's wanted to talk," Richard said, answering the question, but not looking at the questioner. "I'll start a conversation, asking, 'Remember Christie? Remember José?' and he'll talk about them, but he stops short of talking directly and seriously about the fact that they are dead and that they more or less had what he has and what that means for him.

"Once I tried asking what he thought heaven was like. He wouldn't touch that one either. He knows enough to know he doesn't want to know any more."

The room was silent for nearly a minute before Javier spoke up.

"I think we have to talk to him again," he said. "I don't think we can make him DNR without telling him about it. I'm not comfortable with that. I've always explained things to him, and that's why he trusts me. I can't do this behind his back."

"What if he doesn't want to talk?" Kay asked.

"Then maybe he'll listen."

"Can I be there?" she said.

"I would be grateful if both of you could be," Javier said, his glance including both Kay and Richard. It didn't extend to Sally, and she didn't ask why.

"When?" Richard said.

"The sooner the better."

"Tomorrow morning?" offered Kay.

"I'll be free at eleven."

Schedules were checked, the time was good for all of them, and there was nothing left to be said. Javier recapped his pen, and Sally was about to rise from her chair when the door opened, and Oria Dismuke rushed in. She was out of breath, and the hairnet she wore as part of her Hermann cafeteria uniform was coming unpinned in places.

She apologized for being nearly an hour late, blamed it on car trouble, then took a seat, and looked expectantly around the table waiting for the meeting to begin. Sally settled back into her chair. Javier slid his pen back and forth between his forefinger and his thumb and described to Oria in simple language what he planned for Patrick. He was careful to explain that they were not giving up on the boy, that they still cared about him and that they were interested only in his comfort. "More surgery won't work," he said. "It will cause more pain. Shocking his chest if his heart stops won't help him either. He's too weak to survive that for long."

While he spoke, Oria fidgeted. She hates meetings like these. She feels she is being judged, and she is right. She is confused by the medicalese and embarrassed at her shadowy presence in her own baby's life.

Ever since her husband walked out, Oria Dismuke has been the family breadwinner, sometimes working as many as three jobs at a time—a cashier at a school lunchroom, the night cleaning crew at a Houston nursing home, tending the grill at a hospital cafeteria. The money buys the Nintendo games she can't bear to deny her son, but it also means she simply doesn't have time to care for him. Her ramshackle house is next door to her mother's equally worn home, which is where Patrick sleeps when he isn't in the hospital. It is his grandmother, Romania Lewis, whom he has always called "Mom."

Oria does love her son, but she expresses that love—

or, more accurately, fails to express it—in a way that infuriates those who take care of Patrick. She is a large, lumbering woman, and everything about her is slow. She speaks slowly, as if each word is an effort. She moves as if carrying leaden weights. Her son and his problems seem to exhaust her. She is hardly stupid, but sometimes she pretends to be because it is easier. If the doctors think she doesn't understand, she once confessed, perhaps they will stop asking her to make decisions she doesn't want to make.

When she visits Patrick in the hospital, the two often sit in silence, he flipping the television channels with the remote control, she napping in a chair or fixing her graying hair. They rarely talk. This is not a chatty family. She usually leaves after an hour, rarely saying exactly when she will return, and often she isn't seen again for several days. Patrick's chart is filled with snippy notes from the nurses about Oria's behavior on any given day. "Mom might visit but did not want anything said to Patrick in case she doesn't," is one common comment. "Mom visited, slept, left," is another.

What the notes don't say and the nurses don't know is that Oria has decided that the doctors and nurses really are better parents to Patrick than she can ever be. They are more educated, more sophisticated, wealthier, and, most important, they can ease his pain and make him well when she cannot. For more than a decade, there has not been a single day when she had the final word on the basics of his life. She has become accustomed to standing aside and watching while others take over. Her proudest day, she says shyly, was last year, when the social workers arranged for her to work in the cafeteria of Hermann, flipping hamburgers. The hidden agenda of Social Work was that she might visit her son more often if she was just an elevator ride away. It worked (for a while), but not because of the added proximity. The new job meant she wore a Hermann ID badge, finally making her feel more like a part of Patrick's care-taking team.

She was wearing that badge as she listened to Javier explain that Patrick was going to die. While he spoke, she stared at her hands, which fluttered in her lap, and she never met Javier's gaze. For a while, he wasn't sure she was even listening. But when he reached the part about his plans to talk to Patrick, her hands became still, and she looked up slightly, as if she were about to speak. Sally beat her to it.

"I know what you're thinking," she said, remembering her own anguish when her baby daughter died and trying to drag Oria out of an obvious state of denial. "You don't want to face this. But you have to face this. We all do. He has to be told he's going to die. I would sure want to know. I would want that honesty so I could prepare."

Her words hit their mark, but they had a completely unexpected effect. Ever so slowly Oria raised her head and looked Sally straight in the eye. It was a look no one in the room had ever seen before. Then, just as slowly and deliberately, she began to speak. Each word shook with anger and determination, and her listeners were stunned.

"Don't you think he knows?" she said. "Don't you think he already knows? If he wants to talk, he will. I don't have no right to make him talk. You don't neither. This is his way, so it's my way too.

"You can't go and tell my child that. If you tell him how sick he is and that he's dying, then that would just give him a better reason to up and die. Patrick knows it.

Let him deal with it. But don't you go and tell him it's time to give up."

For years, everyone around Patrick had tried to coax Oria to act less like a spectator and more like his mother and to stand her ground when it came to his care. Suddenly, for the first time in hospital memory, she had. And the very people who had so often begged her for her opinion were now sorry they had asked. What Oria Dismuke was raising was a question so complicated that it could easily fill a separate meeting of the Ethics Committee. Technically, Patrick was a minor, and his mother had the right to make decisions for him. But for as long as he could put his foot down, Patrick had insisted on being treated like an adult, and the staff had always been careful to respect his need to know everything that was happening to him. If DNR were explained to him in simple terms, the staff was sure he would understand. So the dilemma posed by Oria was this: It was legal not to tell Patrick of the plan, but was it right?

Javier answered the question without hesitating.

"I promise to respect your wishes," he said. "We won't talk to him about DNR if you tell us not to."

Even as he was speaking he was bothered by his haste. He was so startled by Oria's new assertiveness that he forgot to think first. It was only after the words were out that he realized that keeping his promise would mean hiding the truth from Patrick. In the coming weeks, he would wonder constantly whether he should have taken more time before he spoke.

The meeting broke up quickly after that, with everyone remembering a patient who needed to be seen or a task that simply had to be done. Only Oria lingered, dabbing her eyes with a worn handkerchief and sighing deeply.

After several minutes of silence, she went down the hall to talk to Patrick, who still had a breathing tube stuck down his throat. Unbeknownst to Javier, she even raised the subject of death.

"Pat, do you want to talk about dyin'?" she said to the tiny boy who was playing with Nintendo, refusing to meet her gaze.

He shook his head and scribbled "leave me alone" in crayon on his notepad.

Oria never raised the subject again.

JULY

Armando

Dr. David MacDougall was taking a brief, well-earned nap on a couch in the Neurosurgery Department's conference room when his beeper sounded at 3 A.M. It was the emergency room calling, and the conversation had been brief, a basic recitation of the facts. The patient was a Latin American male, age twenty-four, who had been shot at 1:15 A.M. One bullet had grazed his skull, near his left temple, and the other had entered through the back of the neck where it penetrated the spinal cord. The caliber of the bullet was unknown but, as the surgeon on the other end of the line had joked, "it was certainly big enough to hurt."

The patient had been taken to Madison County hospital in a private car. It was unclear whether he could take any breaths on his own during that trip or what effect the lack of oxygen had on his brain. When he arrived at the hospital, about six minutes after the shooting, he was given CPR and put on a ventilator. After he was stabilized, he was transferred by helicopter to Hermann. As far as anyone in the ER had observed, he couldn't move his arms or legs, but the more detailed exam would be left to David MacDougall.

"He's not going to make it," the caller said. "Except for the gunshot, he's basically healthy. He'll make a good donor."

David hung up the phone and walked quickly down the five flights of stairs between the neurosurgery floor and the emergency room. Even in the middle of the night, taking the stairs at Hermann is faster than waiting for the elevator.

Armando Dimas lay, heavily drugged but somewhat conscious, on a stretcher in the middle of the gleaming room. He looked small for a grown man, about 125 pounds, and he was squinting in the bright overhead lights. A nurse stood at the left side of his stretcher, adjusting the monitors that tracked his heartbeat and respiration rate. An X-ray technician was at the far side of the room, fitting a newly developed picture of Armando's skull into a manila-colored sleeve and placing it next to his chart on a scratched steel table. There was a brown paper bag on the floor with the clothes he had been wearing that evening. They were in shreds where they had been cut from his body by the staff in the emergency room.

A hospital-issue sheet was tucked around him from the rib cage down, but his numerous and dramatic tattoos were fully visible against his pale brown skin. A snarling tiger crouched along his left arm, a sultry woman vamped down the length of his right arm, and a woman, a man, and a flower were sketched randomly across his chest. Colorful, David thought, as he entered the room and saw his patient for the first time.

David leaned over the stretcher so that Armando did not have to turn to see his face. The patient's eyes were open and he looked responsive and alert. The doctor made a mental note, which would soon become a more formal chart entry, that the lack of oxygen did not appear to have made this man a vegetable.

Straightening from his stooped position, he reached for the X-ray envelope and pulled out the films. What he saw made him inhale so sharply, he whistled. The devastation caused by a bullet to the spine depends largely on where it enters the spine. The lower the bullet, the less the damage, because the severed nerves will most likely be below the point of injury. Therefore, a shot to the lumbar region, or the lower back, will likely paralyze the hips and legs, but leave the arms alone. A shot to the thoracic vertebrae, or those in the back of the rib cage, will take the feeling in the chest area, too. A bullet in the cervical vertebrae, which are in the neck, can paralyze everything from the neck down. The opaque sheets that David was holding against a lighted box in the emergency room showed a bullet lodged higher in the spinal cord than he had ever seen before in a patient who had survived. It had entered in the area of the C-3 vertebral segment, near the base of the neck, and traveled upward through the spinal column, where it was plainly visible above the C-1 vertebra, the very first of the cervical vertebrae in the neck. It was so close to the top of that marshmallow-sized piece of bone that it was lodged more or less through the skull and into the back of the brain.

"This guy should be dead," David thought, and slipped the X rays back into their envelope.

For the next fifteen minutes, he conducted a physical exam that would essentially confirm what he already knew. Leaning back over the stretcher he looked at Armando and asked, "Can you hear me?"

The patient didn't move. David looked up at the nurse, still standing at Armando's side. He knew she spoke Spanish, most of the ER nurses do, and his glance was an invitation for her assistance.

"If you can hear me, blink your eyes twice," she said, translating for David. Two blinks, they knew from experience, were less likely to be an accident or a coincidence.

The blinks were weak, but they came one right after the other. If Armando could have smiled, he would have, he was so relieved to have found even the most imperfect way to communicate.

"Follows commands with eye opening and closure," David would later write in the chart.

Through his interpreter he told Armando, "I'm going to ask you some questions then give you four choices as answers. Blink twice at the answer you think is correct."

"What month is it? December?" Armando's eyes stayed open. "May?" Open still. "July?" Two deliberate blinks.

"Where are you now? A restaurant?" No response. "A hospital?" Two blinks.

"What is your name? Armando?" Two blinks, followed by two more for emphasis.

David wrote in the chart: "Oriented to time, person, and place."

Taking a pen light from his pocket, the doctor then shined the narrow beam into Armando's eyes, first the right one and then the left. Each pupil constricted quickly. If there had been swelling in the brain it would probably have blocked the nerve that controls pupillary response. The fast reaction time, coupled with Armando's apparent alertness, led David to believe that this was an injury of the spine only and not the brain. Poor man, he thought, he'll be able to understand what's happened.

Turning back to his patient, the nature of the questions changed.

"Can you move your right leg?" Nothing happened.

"Your left leg?" Nothing.

"Right arm?" Nothing.

"Are you trying right now to move your arm?" Two blinks but no movement.

"Now your left arm." Again, nothing.

"Shrug your shoulders like this." The doctor's shoulders went up and down but Armando's stayed still.

"Turn your head to your right, toward me." The head on the pillow turned ever so slightly.

"Good. Now turn back the other way, away from me." The head moved again.

"Can you furrow your forehead like this?" Armando tried and found that he could.

"Can you wiggle your nose? Very good."

As he went through the familiar game of neurological Simon Sez, David was frustrated. Not with the poor response he was getting—that was hardly the patient's fault—but with the fact that he was doing these tests in the first place. This man had no chance of recovery. Even if he survived, which was unlikely, injuries such as this one do not reverse themselves. In neurosurgery slang, Armando would spend his life as "a head in a bed," with a body that was more or less irrelevant. David felt pity for patients such as these, and he questioned whether it was worth saving a life if it was to be spent trapped in a motionless prison. If CPR hadn't been given at Madison County Hospital, Armando would be dead, not lying on a stretcher under klieg lights, being run through a series of tests he would inevitably fail.

David's is often a depressing line of work, one that involves a lot of diagnosis but relatively little cure. There are some neurosurgery patients who can be made normal again, and they are the ones who drew David to the field. He loves the challenge of examining a patient with a suspected brain lesion, guessing the location of that lesion on the basis of what the patient can and cannot do, then entering the skull with a scalpel and removing the clump of tissue that has changed a personality or crippled an otherwise healthy body.

But severe head and spine injuries don't lend themselves to such white knight solutions, and those injuries are the bulk of a neurosurgeon's work, particularly at a regional trauma center like Hermann. The goal for these patients is incremental progress, not full recovery. Success is the ability to do something that was impossible last week—speak a complete sentence, lift an arm a quarter of an inch higher, tie a pair of shoes. During the five years he had been in training, David had learned to find satisfaction in such incremental progress, and most of the time his relative inability to cure these patients no longer weighed on him when he went home at night. Except for cases like Armando's. He was certain there would be no progress here, yet everything had been done to save this patient, and everything more would be done to keep him alive. Lying on the stretcher, blinking and furrowing, he symbolized to David the new unanswerable question of medicine: How much is too much?

Would I want to be saved for a life like this? David wondered. He answered himself without a pause. Absolutely not.

He reached into the overstuffed pocket of his white lab coat and fished about for one of the safety pins he always carries. He held it at arm's length until it was easily within Armando's field of vision, then he pinched it open as he talked. "I'm going to touch you with the point of this pin," he said. "Blink twice if you feel it."

David started his pinpricking at the point Armando was most likely to have sensation—his forehead, just below the scalp. He pressed the thin stick of metal against the skin with enough pressure to make a fleeting indentation but not enough to draw blood. Armando felt the pain along his forehead, at the tip of his ears, the end of his nose, the center of his ear lobes, and the start of his jaw. When the pin reached his chin, he felt nothing. As far as David could tell, Armando had no sensation and no movement below his ears.

With a quick good-bye to his patient and a promise to see him later, David left the room and spent a few minutes scribbling in the chart.

"No movement of upper or lower extremities," he wrote. "No shoulder shrug. Can turn head side to side slightly, limited by collar. Facial musculature works. Tongue movement noted.

"CAT scan shows bullet fragments entering spinal canal and lodged from C-2 up into the medulla. Should imagine this man will have multiple early complications, particularly pulmonary as well as cardiac regulation. Prognosis for recovery is poor should he survive."

He signed his name on the space for "Consultant's Signature" and stepped out into the hallway to talk to Armando's family. They had almost certainly broken traffic laws and possibly speed records in their race to Hermann from Madisonville. They left for Houston before Armando did, as soon as they learned the chopper was on its way. The drive should have taken nearly three hours, and they made it in less than two. Emergency room doctors often marvel that relatives don't regularly become patients trying to get to the hospital in time.

Once they arrived at Hermann, the Dimas family stayed huddled in a corner of the waiting area across from the emergency room. Armando's mother, looking frail and rigid, sat in a straight-backed chair against the beige cinder-block wall, across from the information counter and next to the gift shop. The years spent raising twelve children showed on her lined, worn face. The hours spent harvesting other people's crops showed in her gnarled, veined hands.

Standing around her, a shield from curious strangers, were four of her twelve children. Her husband, Armando's father, stood several feet away, very separate from the huddled group. As David crossed the waiting area to speak to the family, he took in their body language and felt without question that the mother was the center and the strength of this family and the one he should treat with the most care.

He was right. Victoria Dimas always feared that Armando, her middle child, would meet with trouble, and she had done what she could to stop it. He wasn't a bad boy, she would say, but he had a weakness for bad things. She tried to keep him closer to home, but he would not be controlled. She tried to get his father to be strict where her authority failed, but he did not agree that Armando needed to be tamed. Time would calm his wild streak, he told her. Life would sober him, and he would grow into a good man.

On the day he was shot, Armando had been in the United States for twelve years. He was here illegally, although he and his entire family had applied recently for legal residency under the newly passed amnesty laws. He had arrived in the United States from Matamoros, Mexico, a town that defines poverty. His father was the first to cross the border, and he worked and saved for several years before he sent for his wife and children. They walked together across the Rio Grande, at a point where the river narrows to a trickle, then hitched a ride to Houston, 354 miles to the north. It took three more weeks for them to make their way to the small rural town where their father was working in a mushroom factory, cleaning and stemming the vegetables.

Home for the family of fourteen was a five-room trailer with cracked windows. Armando and four of his brothers shared one cramped bedroom. The heating system in the house never really worked, but the stove usually did, and everyone gathered in the kitchen for warmth during the blessedly short Texas winters. The better life they had moved here to find was always a few paychecks out of reach. Armando had begun the sixth grade in Mexico but only attended school in Madisonville for two weeks. He was suspended for fighting, along with a few of his brothers. He says some other boys started the fight by cursing at his brothers in English, knowing that they spoke only Spanish.

Refusing to return to school, he worked in a restaurant washing dishes and joined his father at the mushroom factory and other grimy agricultural jobs. He saved enough for his first car, a brown 1972 Oldsmobile Cutlass. Shortly after he paid the $500, the engine block cracked, leaving him without savings or transportation.

When he was seventeen, he left home against his mother's protests and ended up in Fort Worth. He had never been there and knew nothing about the city, but he liked the sound of its name. He was planning on seeing the world and Fort Worth was to be his start. He took a job cleaning the trash dumpsters at a construction site. He made doors in a factory. He washed more dishes. He drank often and brawled frequently. He never made more than $150 a week.

He had been in Fort Worth for less than a month when he fell in love with Carolyn Alvarez, a single mother supporting two children with odd jobs and welfare. Her story was much the same as his—her family was originally from Mexico, her childhood had been poor, and she was still living with her parents because she could not afford to strike out on her own. There were two twists to her tale that set it apart from his and that made him think she was blessed where he was merely ordinary. She was born in the United States and she had spent enough time in school to learn to read and write. She wanted to teach him how, but he was proud and impatient and a lousy student. So she did the reading for both.

They lived together for five years, during which time they had a son, Armando, Jr. It was not a great life, but they had two rooms that were theirs as long as the rent was paid and enough money to go to a neighborhood restaurant once in a while or to a movie.

Then, at the beginning of the summer, Armando was laid off from the latest in a series of construction jobs. The pink slip led him to a bar, and the whiskey led him to a fight. Soon, two burly men were after him and he thought it best to leave town. He headed for Madisonville with vague hopes of finding a job in the mushroom factory he swore he would never enter again.

Several months later, on the night he cannot forget, he went with his parents, one of his sisters, and four of his brothers to a party for his niece's first birthday. It was a child's birthday celebration only as an excuse to hold a party. There was no pin the tail on the donkey and no fruit punch or cake. There was abundant tequila and tobacco, however, and Armando was soon having a very good time.

Shortly after midnight, the beer ran out, and when a drunken guest asked Armando for a drink, Armando filled an empty whiskey bottle with water and handed it to the man. Like a scene from an old Western, the man took a sip, realized he was being fooled, and spat the water at Armando. Then he issued a wobbly challenge to a fight. The man swung a punch that met only air. Armando responded by beating the man with a chair. Two gunshots were fired—Armando could not figure out who fired them—and the party broke up. Armando never even caught the man's name.

The Dimas family left the party at 1 A.M., and began to walk home. Armando walked ahead with three of his brothers. His mother and father walked several yards behind. About fifteen minutes later, when they were two trailer lots away from their own home, Armando saw the man appear from behind a bush, raise a gun and fire twice, hitting Armando both times. The man fled and was never found.

Armando remembers nothing after that. His mother remembers everything. The lift from a neighbor to the emergency room, where they wouldn't let her see her son for the longest time. The doctor in the white coat, too clean, she thought, for this dirty job, who came to tell her that Armando might die. He said a helicopter was coming to take him to another hospital, one she never heard of, in Houston, a big city that she didn't like. The doctor said that, if Armando died, someone would ask her about donating his heart and other parts of his body and that she should start to think about that now. The ride to Houston, filled with tears, prayers, and short exhausted naps. The wait in the visiting area with no one to explain what was happening.

Then, suddenly, another doctor approached her, a tall, blond man, very young, with a friendly face, also wearing a white coat. She was sure he had come to tell her that her son was dead and to ask her about his organs. Instead, he extended his hand and introduced himself as Dr. David MacDougall. He talked about Armando as if he were still alive.

"I'm sure you already understand that he has incurred

a devastating injury," David said through a translator, this time a member of the Patient Relations staff. "We can't be certain whether or not he will survive. There could be many complications during the next few days that could kill him, and you have to understand that."

Experience told him to leave his explanation brief. He felt he only had their attention for a limited time, and there was a lot of information to give before the crying and denial began.

"As far as the long-term prognosis," he continued, "the bullet entered near the back of his neck. Rather than remain outside the spinal column it went into the spinal cord and tracked upward, into what's called the brainstem. As it traveled upward, it tore the spinal cord, and it just happened to lodge in the very worst place. It was too low to kill him, which is good. It was also too low to affect his brain function. But it was high enough to eliminate all spinal function from the point of entry on down."

Seeing the look of confusion on Mrs. Dimas's face, David tried an analogy. "If I gave you a gun with one bullet and told you to knock out all the lights in this hospital, you wouldn't shoot at just this bulb," he said, pointing toward the fluorescent fixture above their heads. "You would go to the switchbox. Well, this bullet hit the switchbox."

"It's likely that he's not going to walk again. I can't tell you never, but I do think that it's very unlikely. On rare occasions a patient can be in spinal shock, and the lack of feeling and motion can be due to swelling or shock, and it can eventually reverse. I've never seen it happen, but theoretically it could."

While he talked, the family sat silently and listened. David had seen their expression before. They weren't hearing most of what he was saying, and much of what they did hear, they didn't understand. But he knew they wouldn't ask him to repeat or explain anything. Not yet. All they could do now was let his carefully phrased sentences wash over them, as if the words themselves had a cleansing, soothing effect. He paused for a moment to give them a chance to speak, and Mrs. Dimas's question confirmed that she had barely taken in one word.

"Is he in pain?" she asked.

David resisted any urge to point out that it was the lack of pain that was her son's problem and if he could feel his wounds, he would be better off.

"Not that I can tell," David answered. "He is uncomfortable because of the breathing tube, and the cut on his forehead probably stings, but he doesn't seem to be in any pain."

"When will he be able to walk?" Mrs. Dimas asked.

"We don't think that he will be, but I promise we will tell you if there is any change," he said, realizing that this conversation would have to take place again in a few hours or days. He thanked the translator for her help, briefly took Mrs. Dimas's hand, then walked away.

First we have to see if he's going to live, he thought, as he stepped through the emergency room doors.

The Committee

Lin Weeks's office is an average-sized hospital administrator's box, with room for a desk, a bookcase, two filing cabinets, and a small round table. The cabinets are packed with years of medical research papers, most of which she has actually read. The bookcase is crammed with texts on organizational paradigms, nursing techniques, ethical theory, and the book she wrote herself, *Advanced Cardiovascular Nursing*. The table can seat only three people—two if they want to be comfortable.

The desk is strewn with pictures of the man in her life and Xeroxed witty sayings. Her favorite is from Carl Sandburg, a list titled "The Four Stumbling Blocks to the Truth." On the list are: "The influence of fragile and unworthy authority ... Custom ... The imperfection of undisciplined senses ... Concealment of ignorance by ostentation of seeming wisdom."

Her secretary, Ellen Nuñez, adds a stack of mail to the cluttered desk each day, making sure to slit open each envelope and smooth the contents flat, tossing the obvious junk mail as she goes. The resulting pile is usually a mixture of interoffice memos and glossy medical journals, but one morning, a few weeks after her Ethics Committee discussed Patrick, a short handwritten note caught Lin's attention. It was from a twenty-seven-year-old woman named Teresa Knepper, an Exxon engineer who had no medical training and had never worked in a hospital but who wanted to join the Hermann Ethics Committee.

With her chin in her fist and her elbow on her desktop, Lin read the letter several times. She was intrigued. Lin is forever tinkering with her committee, adding an obstetrician here, a neonatologist there, as though she could find a perfect version that would be all-wise and all-compassionate if only she fiddled long enough. The fine-tuning energizes her. A literal student of hospital bureaucracy (she is working for her doctorate in health service organization), she is constantly toying—on paper, at least—with traditional hospital structure. Although she can gossip and make small talk with the best of them, she gets *really* excited when discussing books that change her understanding of how hospitals work.

On some people this would be stuffy, but on Lin it is endearing and infectious. A trim, athletic woman, with close-cropped blond hair and a peach glow to her skin, she leans forward when she talks, locking eyes with her listener. As she warms to her subject, her hands move almost as rapidly as her lips, waving a pen, a paper clip, or whatever else is handy. Ever efficient, she keeps her sentences clipped and short, often trailing off with nonsense sounds, like "da, da, da, da, da, da," leaving the listener to fill in the blanks as she moves on to the next animated thought.

A lot of those thoughts are of illness and death. For a healthy woman in her forties, Lin spends an unusual amount of time thinking about both. She is not afraid of dying. What she is afraid of is not having any control over the way she dies. She has read widely about old Indian cultures where elders say good-bye to their families one morning and walk calmly into the forest, knowing that their time has come. Today, those same elders would probably linger on a respirator in the care of a doctor they had never met.

Lin doesn't want her life to end like that, with no one willing to turn off a machine that is merely postponing her death. At some hospitals, her wishes would be honored, but at others the inertia of the bureaucracy would get in the way. Policies, designed to prevent lawsuits, would be unbendable. Doctors, unaccustomed to thinking about death as anything but the enemy, would be unwilling to listen to her request.

She watched it happen in her own family in a hospital several miles from Hermann one recent Christmas Eve. A sudden and violent case of pneumonia left her mother in an irreversible coma, and doctors refused to disconnect the tubes that kept her breathing. Lin knew that her mother's greatest fear was that she would end up like her own mother, who had lost all control over her mind after a stroke.

"She wouldn't have wanted it like this. She made us promise she would never live on a machine," Lin told the doctor.

"There's nothing we can do," the doctor said. "Hospital policy."

It took tears and the threat of legal action before the machine was unplugged, and to Lin, her mother's undignified death was a failure of modern medicine, which makes it easier to continue care than to stop it. Part of her commitment to the Hermann Ethics Committee is born of determination that what happened to her mother not happen to anyone else.

Lin had been chairman of the Ethics Committee for only a year on the morning she received the note suggesting Teresa as a member, but she had been involved with the committee since it began in 1983. Like other committees around the country, the Hermann committee is a response to the new realities of health care: legal fears, moral uncertainty, a need to codify policy, the fact that the daily questions of medicine have gotten harder. Respirators, for instance, were unheard of in hospitals until the late 1950s and were not universally used for years after that. In vitro fertilization is a product of the 1980s, and heart transplants were not common until 1982, when the antirejection drug cyclosporine was introduced.

It follows that until there are respirators, there can't be a controversy over whether or not to turn those respirators off. Without in vitro fertilization, there can be no debate about what to do with the unused fertilized eggs. Until transplants are possible, there is no question of which of two dying patients should receive the one available heart. The more expensive the technology, the higher the bill and the more heated the debate over who pays it. The tougher the decision, the more complex the decision-making process.

In late 1983, all this weighed heavy on the Reverend Julian Byrd, the head chaplain at Hermann, who, despite his twelve-hour days, felt he wasn't doing enough to help the hospital's patients and their families. When bedside monitors started buzzing and teams of doctors and nurses came running, he always felt somewhat helpless and in the way. What he had to offer— emotional and spiritual support—was not really needed during dramatic medical moments. But it *was* needed during all the decisions that might lead to or result from those moments. He had read of a few hospitals that had ethics committees, and he decided to form one at Hermann.

Among the dozen members he recruited was Lin Weeks. For several months, the small group discussed ethics only in the theoretical sense. They developed a list of committee bylaws and a statement of purpose, but they didn't hear a case. Then one morning in October of 1984, Randy Gleason, the hospital's lawyer, arrived at a meeting with the tale of a seventy-three-year-old woman who had peripheral vascular disease. The circulation to one leg was so poor that the leg would have to be cut off. She refused the operation, and her doctor asked Randy for his opinion. The Ethics Committee was in business.

The central issue in the case was whether the woman was competent to make such a decision. Her doctors thought she wasn't. Lin found herself arguing with a tentative committee that the woman had the right to decide her own fate.

"Doctors have a tendency—and it's not just limited to doctors—to believe that a person's choice is somehow wrong if it is not the choice that the doctor would make," she said.

"If someone says, 'I don't want to have my leg amputated because yesterday little green men came down and told me not to do it,' then that person's incompetent," she continued, her voice surprisingly soft given the sharpness of her words. "However, if they say, 'I don't want to have my leg cut off because I'm seventy-three and I've lived a full life, my health's bad, and I don't want to have the further problem of living the rest of my life in a debilitated condition,' that patient is not incompetent. That is what we have to get across to everybody."

She did, and ten days later the woman died, at home, in her own bed.

The Reverend Mr. Byrd left Hermann Hospital in 1987 to form an ethics committee down the block at Methodist Hospital, and Lin Weeks became chairman of the Hermann committee.

The Hermann Hospital Ethics Committee is large—twenty-three members—and growing at the rate of one every other month. That number is a bit unwieldy, but Lin believes it's necessary if it is to include representatives of all the major subspecialties in the hospital. She doesn't have all of them yet, but the list does include doctors from at least a dozen areas of expertise (with a heavy representation of neonatologists, like Taylor's doctor, Sharon Crandell, and pediatricians, like Patrick's doctor, Javier Aceves), a full-time ethicist, several nurses, a minister, a priest, and a rabbi, a few social workers, the head of Patient Relations, the head of quality assurance, and the hospital lawyer.

One result of the large size is that the members never become completely at ease with each other, since scheduling conflicts insure that the same combination of people rarely meets twice. Lin has come to think of this as an advantage, though. The feeling of a collegial club would be inappropriate for her committee. Better that everyone be a little bit on edge.

Like most ethics committees around the country, this group has policy meetings. At Hermann they are held the last Friday of every month, from 3:30 P.M. to 4:30 P.M., in the Birch Room, which is across from the emergency room and next to the cafeteria. At these meetings, members sit around a horseshoe-shaped table, sip cans of soda that they fish from a vat of half-melted ice, nibble cheese and fruit, and act like an average hospital committee. They read the minutes of the last session, form subcommittees, worry whether their budget will cover needed Xeroxing costs, and revise their latest policy proposal.

Unlike many ethics committees, however, the Hermann group goes one step further by holding case consultations (in medical jargon these are known as "consults" with the emphasis on the first syllable).

If Hermann's ethicists once worried about the dangers of voting on life and death, they stopped several years ago. Ethics committees run counter to everything Americans idealize medicine to be—personalized, private, and one-on-one, a doctor and patient who have known each other for years, facing life and death together. But that hasn't been the reality of medicine for a long time. In the real world, doctors oversee the deaths of relative strangers, courts step in to second-guess both sides, and some of the most important medical decisions are made in groups.

Over the years, Lin and the other members of the Hermann Ethics Committee have become resigned to that reality. So sporadically, and with little advance notice, they gather in Room 3485 for the periodic case consults, such as the one about Patrick. Whereas the monthly business meetings are chatty and relaxed, the consults are tense and unpredictable, with everyone acting a little less like committee members and a little more like individuals asked to decide the impossible, each one dealing with the burden in his own way.

Anyone can ask the group for a consult, including a doctor or nurse on the case, a social worker, the patient, the patient's family, even an outside observer who feels a situation is being mishandled, though that has never happened here. The most common scenario is when a family questions a doctor's treatment. About half the time, the doctor decides that nothing more can be done, and the family insists that the doctor isn't being aggressive enough. Half the time it's the other way around, the family wants to withdraw care, and the doctor refuses. Often, some family members agree with the doctor, and others disagree.

Whatever the origins of the dispute, someone calls Lin Weeks, who asks her secretary to reserve a meeting room and assemble a quorum of six. Usually the patient is too sick to attend—that, after all, is why the hearing is necessary in the first place—but the family is invited. Here the feelings of the family count, and the patient is more than just the sum of his age, sex, race, and symptoms. The committee asks the family questions: Tell us about your son/daughter/mother/father/husband/wife. Help us to know in fifteen minutes what you have learned in years. Convince us that they would/wouldn't want this treatment/surgery/decision to turn off the machine. We know this isn't ideal, but it's the only thing we have. Do you need a Kleenex? I'm sorry, we have none.

After the questions are asked, the family and other noncommittee members leave the room while the group makes its decision. That is standard procedure at Hermann, on the theory that the privacy of a hearing room allows members to give their opinions freely. Aware that this smacks of a jury rendering its verdict, members nonetheless defend the process, pointing out that jury decisions are binding whereas committee decisions are not. Officially, the committee only gives consultation and advice, which the parties are free to reject. The advice is almost always followed.

That scares a lot of doctors, many of whom will not bring cases to the committee and who talk among themselves about the self-important group that is trying to take intimate decisions even further from the bedside. It scares Lin, too, which is why she is always fine-tuning her committee, adding members from as many divisions as she can. She realizes the power of the group, and it makes her nervous. She distrusts any committee, even if it is her own, and every so often something will remind her how easy it is for her group to become isolated and smug, insular and out of touch, at a safe distance from the raw emotions of the patient. At those times, she wonders if a complete outsider might add some needed perspective and sensitize the committee to how it feels to be a patient. The letter about Teresa was one of those reminders.

Teresa Knepper certainly knows all about being a patient. In 1981 she was nineteen years old, newly married, and a chemical engineering student at the University of Florida at Gainesville when her twins were born three months before they were due. They weighed 2½ pounds apiece at birth, nearly twice the size of Jake and Taylor Poarch, but that advantage did not protect Mark, the younger, who died after two days. The added size did help Matthew, however, and he came home after nearly three months in intensive care. He was so tiny, his homecoming outfit fit one of his mother's childhood dolls.

Getting Matthew out of intensive care would be only the first hurdle for Teresa and her husband, David. The baby's first year was a nightmare. He screamed constantly, arched his spine, and tried to throw himself backward until Teresa thought her child might actually be possessed. Her constant calls to the doctor brought little insight or reassurance, but they did result in a house call from the infant development team at the hospital where he was born. The two traveling social workers came loaded with exercise routines Teresa had to learn and color-coded charts she had to fill out to prove she was following instructions. The social workers seemed certain the problem was that this mother didn't know how to comfort her son, and they showed her how to swaddle him in blankets when he became upset. The only effect Teresa could see was that the swaddling made Matthew scream even louder.

The pressure of caring for a hysterical infant while

being told she was doing it all wrong took its understandable toll on Teresa's nerves. When she started daydreaming about ending her constant feelings of helplessness by wrapping her car around a tree, Teresa started seeing a psychiatrist. Her marriage suffered too. David Dyal is sixteen years older than his wife, and their different ways of dealing with the baby were as disparate as their ages. While Teresa clung fiercely to Matthew, her husband distanced himself, convinced that the child was mentally retarded and didn't need a father's love.

As David is now the first to admit, that prediction was wrong. Matthew is not mentally retarded. But he does have cerebral palsy, which was not diagnosed until he was more than a year old. Because of his condition, he had never learned the simplest of baby achievements. He could not crawl, walk, talk, or even roll over except as an involuntary side effect of a spasm in his back. He was not able to hold a bottle or a toy, and even sucking, one of the instincts in human newborns, was difficult for him. He was still on formula months after others his age were eating solid food, and Teresa began to cut the bulbs off the nipples of his bottles so she could, in her words, "just pour it in him."

It took more than a year for her pediatrician to conclude that all this was due to cerebral palsy, a permanent disorder of the neurons that control the muscles. Teresa was relieved. It meant she wasn't crazy and that she wasn't a bad mother, either. For the first time, she felt like Matthew was her child. Until then, she had felt he really belonged to the visiting social workers and that she was simply caring for him indefinitely. Now her house calls were by a physical therapist familiar with cerebral palsy who quickly concluded that the worst thing for the baby was stimulation of his overly sensitive back muscles. Swaddling put pressure on those muscles, so did cradling him with an arm along his back, as Teresa had been doing. When he was held backward, in effect, with her hand around his stomach, he immediately calmed down.

Soon he showed he understood what was being said around him, even laughing at his mother's jokes. He will never be able to walk, but he did learn to crawl by dragging himself with his hands. He learned to talk when he was three years old, and will always be difficult to understand. With his first attempts at words, his father's defensive wall melted, and they have become great friends.

When Matthew was two, Teresa was invited to join the ethics committee of Shands Teaching Hospital in Gainesville, Florida, where she had spent so many frantic hours while her son was in intensive care. She was intimidated at first, but the small committee patiently explained adult diseases and dilemmas just as the nurses had explained about Matthew. She read stacks of articles, anything she could find, on medical ethics and every disease that came before the committee.

During the three years she sat on the committee, she often talked about her son. When she thought a doctor was too quick to criticize a patient's family, she told the story of the social workers who turned out to be wrong. When she thought a patient's quality of life was being dismissed too lightly, she described her own child, using much the same words and the same fervent tone every time.

"He's happy because he doesn't know any other way," she would say. "He knows he has cerebral palsy but he doesn't weep about it. He thinks he's normal, and all the other kids have a problem. He doesn't look longingly at the children in the playground and wish he could do that. I may want to have long blond hair, but I can live without it. No one has every single thing they want in life."

The other members didn't always agree with her, but she gained their respect. In the fall of 1987, after she had graduated and was about to start a job with Exxon in Houston, she was called for one last emergency consult. When she arrived, she found the meeting was really a surprise going-away party. She still uses the leather attaché case that was her parting gift.

Her pediatrician in Florida sent her to Javier Aceves in Houston, Patrick's doctor. During a meeting with Javier's nurse, Sally Olsen, Teresa mentioned her work at Shands Hospital and Sally suggested that she join the committee at Hermann. Teresa sent a note to Lin, who called Teresa, heard her story, and invited her to become the first nonmedical, nonclerical member of the Hermann Ethics Committee.

Taylor

Houston, so the wisecrack goes, is a very good place to get very, very sick. There are sixty-five hospitals in and around the city, and the densest concentration of those is in the Texas Medical Center. From an airplane, its skyline rivals the one in downtown Houston—not as flashy, perhaps, but as impossible to miss. The Med Center's 526 acres are crammed with fifty buildings that house fourteen hospitals, two medical schools, four nursing schools, and assorted rehabilitation facilities, research labs, libraries, and doctors' offices. More than 55,000 people are paid to work here, and thousands more students labor for free. The center generates more than $3 billion for the local economy each year.

Even at the nadir of the oil bust, there were still construction cranes on the streets of the medical center—the only place in the city where there was building going on. The entire complex has the feeling of a city set apart, bunkered from the outside world by a series of underground passages and aerial walkways, all air-conditioned against the brutal Houston summers.

This minicity even has its own monthly newspaper, the *Medical Center News*, and two separate private police forces. The officers spend most of their time jump-starting cars, but, if necessary, they have full legal power to make arrests. A private bus service crisscrosses the center, connecting the hospitals with each other and with nearby housing complexes. Nearly every drugstore in Houston gives discounts to doctors for their personal purchases. A child-care center, subsidized by many of the hospitals, opens before dawn and closes after midnight, to accommodate the strange hours of hospital staff. Bookstores carry some best-sellers and endless shelves of lesser known works such as *DNA Cloning: A Practical Approach*, and *Speedy Spanish for Physical Therapists*.

Everywhere there are people in baggy scrubs—those unisex outfits that look like pajamas and are favored by doctors and nurses during particularly messy jobs. The scrubs are provided by the hospitals and are stamped with their name and logo. But because the major institutions all use the same laundry service—another civic function performed by the Medical Center—some shuffling inevitably occurs. The woman on line at the supermarket, the one wearing St. Luke's scrubs, may really work at Texas Children's Hospital.

There is a pecking order of scrubs within each hospital. At Hermann, for instance, solid cranberry clothing or a mix of cranberry and white are worn only by licensed nurses in the nurseries. A white-on-white outfit announces "nursing student" almost as clearly as if it were written across the back. Respiratory therapists wear deep blue. The shade with status is sea green, reserved for those who work in sterile areas and for the doctors. Medical students can wear green, but usually with a white jacket affixed with an orange and white badge to make sure they aren't taken too seriously.

Outnumbering the staff are the patients—more than 2 million of them each year, many from Houston, but most from someplace else. They come to have their clogged arteries bypassed, their premature babies incu-

bated, their cancers bombarded, their bodies repaired.
Not all of them stay in the hospital. Many stay nearby,
moving from their hometowns to furnished apartments
here and stopping by the Medical Center daily or
weekly for outpatient care. Perhaps the only thing they
have in common is that they would rather be someplace
else.

They, too, have transformed the community. Local
ambulance services make regular trips to the airport to
pick up incoming patients. The Marriott Hotel in the
medical center has rooms set aside for wheelchair patients. The chef in the Marriott's restaurant is used to
being asked to eliminate all the salt and sugar and butter
from any given dish.

And the patients, too, have their own uniforms. For
some it is the Heplock they wear on their wrists—a
semipermanent tube that dangles from a vein so that a
new hole need not be punched in the arm for each dose
of intravenous drugs. For others it is the white plastic
face mask they wear to prevent catching yet something
else while they take their prescribed walk each evening.
It can be a brace or a cane or a rubber ball carried and
squeezed hundreds of times a day to strengthen a once
useless hand. No matter what their uniform, most seem
to carry pictures or mementos of a time before they
wore it. They share the photos with the acquaintances
they meet at the hospital, a gesture that says, "I had a
normal life once. I wasn't always this way."

Dazed and exhausted, Fran and Carey Poarch joined
this medical world. They had buried Jake in a tiny casket lined with blue-and-white-checked gingham. Carey
wrote and delivered his son's eulogy, choking at a quote
by James Hastings that had come in a sympathy card
from a friend: "The needle that pierces may carry a
thread that binds us to heaven."

Every day since then they had come to see Taylor at Hermann. Fran would wake up early, walk the dog, straighten the house, then drive to the hospital. Doctors' rounds were between ten and noon, and no visitors were allowed during those hours, so she would take walks around the medical center, eating lunch, buying baby clothes six times Taylor's size and trying to lose the weight she had gained while she was pregnant. Then she would return to the hospital and sit with Taylor all day. Carey would join her after work, on weekends, and whenever the baby's condition took a frightening turn. They would make the long drive home at 10 P.M., fall into bed, and begin again the next day.

At first they thought they would never get used to the world that had enveloped Taylor. The Isla Carroll Sterling Turner Neonatal Intensive Care Unit is almost impossible to find if you don't already know where to look. It is located on the third floor of the Robertson Pavilion, down corridors, around corners, and through doorways and on an entirely different floor from the regular nursery. For that, Fran and Carey were grateful. They would have crumpled emotionally if they had been forced to pass a window of healthy babies every time they came to see their daughter.

There are no picture windows onto Turner. There is no way to see inside without actually entering, and the only authorized visitors are parents and grandparents, although those rules can be bent. Turner is designed for the tiniest, most fragile babies, most of whom would have died as recently as five years ago. The nursing ratio is one to one.

Several feet beyond the swinging entrance doors, there is a thick red stripe on the floor, a borderline in the linoleum. No one is allowed to cross that line without scrubbing his or her hands first. For those who forget, there is a detailed sign: "Before you visit your infant remove all jewelry and scrub to elbows with brush for two minutes."

The result is a ritual for entering Turner, almost a religious rite, in which parents purify themselves before visiting their miracle children. The sink is stocked with brushes that are filled with iodine solution in the factory before being wrapped in sterile foil packets. These EZ Scrub Sponge Brushes are dual action, with a soft yellow sponge on one side and sharp white bristles on the other for digging under the nails. The iodine stings a little when it hits the skin. It's not real pain, just a tingling reminder that it's there.

The nurses scrub dozens of times each day, both before and after they touch a patient. None of them wear a watch, which are superfluous anyway because of the dozen or more huge clocks that decorate the walls around the room. They don't wear wedding rings, either, because the metal can't really be sterilized by scrubbing and because the constant exposure to iodine would mottle the gold. The married staff members are the ones with rings dangling from their hospital identification badges.

Once visitors are allowed to enter, they find themselves standing at an island of desks in the center of a circular room. The pillar in the middle of the desks holds a huge map of Texas covered with an opaque set of concentric colored circles radiating from Houston. Each band of color represents 25 miles, and the map is used to prepare for premature babies who are born at outlying hospitals and brought by LifeFlight to Hermann. By knowing the rate at which a helicopter flies—and everyone in this room does—they know how long it will be between the phone call from any outlying hospital and the baby's entrance into their care.

There are chairs at this island of desks, but they are only sporadically used, more often by the medical residents than by the nurses. If there is sitting to be done—feeding the rare baby strong enough to suck from a bottle, for instance—it is done in the half dozen rocking chairs scattered around the room. They are huge wooden pieces of furniture, each with a brass plaque that expresses the thanks of the family who gave it as a gift. Many are dedicated to certain nurses. Others give thanks to everyone. One carries a poem:

> *When I needed help you were there.*
> *When I needed care, you cared.*
> *I hope that when others are in despair,*
> *They too find the love that was built into this chair.*
> *God bless you, Christopher John Peavey.*

The real activity at Turner takes place in the beds that stand perpendicular to the wall with a large number painted over each one. Until ten years ago, the neonatal nursery was one of the quietest places in the hospital because there was so little that could be done. Now, it is one of the busiest. Usually, all of the dozen beds in Turner are full.

The actual beds don't really resemble beds at all; they look more like equipment carts. The largest babies, those closest to the size of a child born at term, do have regular cribs, but it is unusual to see a baby that big in this room. Much warmer than the cribs—and warmth is an important factor when you're born too soon—are the isolettes. They resemble Plexiglas hutches, like a carrying case for a pet, but with gloved portholes instead of airholes so the staff can reach through and check, change, and care.

The isolettes would be ideal if so many preemies

were not connected to ventilators. The breathing machines need constant care that cannot be given in so constrained a case. So Taylor and most of her neighbors lay on neonatal warmers, which are cream and blue carts with tiny mattresses on top and drawers below for supplies. On all four sides of the mattress are Plexiglas walls, about six inches high and rimmed with colored tape so they are visible. The tops of the warmers are waist high on an adult, so the staff need not bend to check on a baby. Above each mattress is a heat lamp, which gives the warmer its name. It is not a bright light, just a warm one. Each bed is also equipped with two temperature monitors, one for the mattress and one for the baby, and an alarm that rings if either reading dips too low.

Each morning when Fran arrived, Taylor lay as he had the night before, in the center of the warmer. As with all preemies, her head was much too large for her body, like an orange on limbs of popsicle sticks. She had not yet developed a protective layer of fat, and her deep blue veins were clearly visible beneath her skin. Her fragile appearance was made more so by the thicket of tubes that surrounded her. Most jarring was the rigid plastic ventilator tube inserted in her mouth and into her lungs, held in place with two pieces of adhesive tape, the first arching over her top lip and the second curving under her bottom lip. The result resembled a white clown's smile. With each puff of the ventilator her chest wall pulsed out and then in again. Two thin plastic tubes were threaded into what would be her belly button once the rest of her umbilical cord fell off. One tube delivered nutrition and medication. The other provided easy access for periodic blood samples needed throughout each day.

On her chest were two electrodes, one that measured

her heart rate and the other her respiration rate. On her abdomen was still another electrode, called a transcutaneous oxygen monitor, or a TCO2, which measured the amount of oxygen passing through the skin. The tiny round disk was heated slightly and had to be moved every few hours to prevent serious burns on her paper-thin skin. Even with those precautions, however, she sometimes had pale red spots on her stomach where the electrode rested a little too long.

It took several weeks, but Fran and Carey gradually got used to the structure and machinery of Turner. Eventually, they could enter the room without the shiver of panic they felt in the early days, and with time they stopped whispering and tiptoeing while they were there. The neonatal ICU became just another familiar place, like the office or the library.

Over time they began to notice the soft touches in the sterile room, gentle reminders that these translucent creatures really are babies, a thought that can be comforting and heartbreaking at the same time. Although flowers were not allowed in the presence of such delicate lungs, there are balloons bobbing over many of the Lilliputian beds, announcing, "It's a Girl," or, "It's a Boy." Mirrors are propped in the corner of some of the isolettes so the bigger babies can see themselves. Pictures of waiting families are taped on the outside of the Plexiglas warmer walls, facing in.

The stethoscopes are tiny, smaller than the ones children use to play doctor. The round plastic patches that attach heart monitor wires to the chest are yellow and are decorated with happy faces. And the scale to measure urine output by weighing the used diapers is appropriately named the Pee Wee Scale.

The nurses talk to their patients as they work. "Good morning, pumpkin, how are we feeling?" "You know you're pretty cute." "Yeah, that ouches. This really stinks, doesn't it?"

Fran immersed herself in this gentler side of Turner. Every day she would read to Taylor, usually fairy tales that she had loved as a child. She bought every stuffed animal she could find and surrounded her daughter with ducks, clowns, rabbits, elephants, and Paddington Bear, dressed like a doctor who wore a sign saying, "My name is Dr. Paddington, and I'm here to take care of Taylor." The smaller animals could share the baby's mattress and the larger ones were sent to sit by the window or on the supply cart, often showing up in drawers meant for cotton balls and skin lotions.

For a change of pace, Fran also purchased every variety of eensy baby socks and matching bows, since real clothing was out of the question until Taylor doubled, if not tripled, her size. Every morning the tiny infant was dressed in matching accessories, a job the nurses adored.

Fran was the first to admit that her doting was not motivated only by love. There was also guilt, anger, isolation, and fear. The guilt came because, as hard as she and Carey might try, they did not think of Taylor as their daughter. She was precious to them, and they quickly built their world around her, but they didn't dare to fantasize about themselves as a family— Taylor's first Christmas, her high school graduation, her wedding, her own firstborn. "I've never had a daughter, so I really don't know how it feels," Fran said. "But I think it should feel different than this."

That guilt came hand in hand with anger. The outrage that Fran had felt in the helicopter, the feelings of why-is-this-happening-to-me? only intensified with each day that she spent at Turner. One month after Jake died, she and Carey attended a support group for the parents of preemies. As a sympathetic film flickered at the front of the room, Fran stared at one mother in the group, a fourteen-year-old girl whose baby, born less than a month early, was to be released that day. She felt rage at the young mother, and she barely heard a word of the film or the discussion afterward. "It's not fair," she said to Carey during their drive home that night. "We go by the book, and she has a healthy baby."

In some ways, the isolation was the toughest to bear. Overnight, Hermann and Taylor became Fran and Carey's entire world. There were no dinners with friends, few telephone calls just to chat, no movies, almost no television, only occasional newspapers. There wasn't even time, Fran realized months later, to mourn for Jake. Every spare moment and ounce of energy was spent worrying about their little girl. They could share this single-minded existence with their parents and the rest of their immediate families, but even that small circle became suffocating. Because only parents and grandparents are allowed to visit babies in Turner, none of Fran's closest friends had ever seen the baby that had taken Fran away from them. Her best friend called less and less often, then stopped altogether and waited for Fran to make the calls. This might happen, Fran and Carey were warned during the support group, but they were too distracted at the time to understand.

Lost for a way to fight the isolation, the new parents burrowed into Hermann all the more. Often they would stay overnight in the conference room across from Turner. Eventually, the staff scheduled meetings elsewhere because the Poarches had practically moved in.

They felt safe in the conference room. Someone had worked hard to make the windowless box as soothing and inviting as possible, knowing that it would often serve as more than just a meeting room. The walls are a warm peach and a peach and beige Oriental rug lies over the institutional brown carpet. The serviceable beige couches are slightly worn, and the pillows are usually piled on one end by a visitor trying in vain to get some sleep. The glass and brass tables hold lacquered Japanese lamps, and one wall is decorated with a Japanese screen of a ship pulling into port. On the opposite wall is a sepia and white drawing of a family, two parents and four daughters, the youngest of whom is still an infant. The baby is being held in her mother's arms, and the woman's chin is nestled on the baby's forehead. Fran would stare at the picture for hours, wondering how it would feel to hold Taylor and take her away from this place.

Over the weeks, the nurses began to worry about Taylor's parents almost as much as they worried about Taylor. Particularly Virginia Lennox. A self-described "baby nut" who had wanted to be a nurse ever since she began her baby-sitting career in grade school, Virginia had been out of nursing school for one year and at Hermann for six months when she met Taylor. She quickly fell in love. It wasn't the first time she had become completely attached to a baby in her care. It had happened in nursing school, too, every six months or so. With the first few babies she tried to pull away, because she knew the inevitable future pain involved, but that never worked, and eventually she just let herself fall.

She couldn't predict which of the babies would latch on to her emotions. Sometimes they looked like a tiny version of someone she knew, sometimes it was a funny expression they would involuntarily make, or a gritty determination to live despite predictions that they would not. With Taylor, it was those eyes. There was a wise personality behind her eyes, and Virginia felt she could communicate with the baby just by looking at her. The big blue eyes had tiny wrinkles around the corners making Taylor look like she was smiling whenever her eyes were open.

Although Virginia had become used to this fierce attachment to some babies, she was startled by the equally strong attachment she developed to Fran and Carey. Some nights she nursed the parents emotionally nearly as much as she nursed the child physically. One weekend, when the couple had spent two anxious days and nights in the peach-walled conference room, Virginia found Carey pacing the halls while Fran was inside trying to sleep. Asking another nurse to watch Taylor, Virginia took Carey down to the cafeteria for a cup of coffee and some advice.

"You have to take care of yourselves," she said, realizing there were some at the hospital who would think it was not a nurse's place to give such advice. "You have to take care of Fran. She can't handle much more of this. You have to get her out of here."

The next night the couple went for a quiet dinner away from Hermann, then drove home to sleep in their own bed.

Fran and Carey were amazed that the nurses were so kind to them. "I'm a pain in the neck," a bewildered Fran told her mother. "I'm a terror when it comes to Taylor. I'm always telling them, 'She does not look comfortable. This does not look right.' When her lips get chapped, I make them bring me lotion and gauze so I can wipe them. Then I stand there and cry because she can't even lick her own lips because of the ventilator. It's such a little thing and she can't do it. So I cry and demand more lotion, and they're all nice to me anyway."

The nurses were oddly pleased by the demands made

by Carey and Fran. They liked these parents because they were smart and caring, the way Taylor's caretakers imagined they would be if their own children were, heaven forbid, in Turner. Parents such as the Poarches are the ever more rare exception in the neonatal ICU, the nurses say. Every year more babies in the isolettes and warmers are those born to prostitutes and IV drug abusers, or to teenagers who didn't know, or didn't want to admit, that they were pregnant and received no pre-natal care. In that way, the patients in Turner reflect na-tional statistics. In some inner-city hospitals, 30 percent of neonatal intensive care babies are born to mothers who use crack or other drugs that induce premature la-bor.

Sometimes the tiny cribs have court orders attached to them prohibiting a parent from visiting the baby. When Taylor arrived at Turner, another baby had just died. The little boy was born several months too soon, the result of a beating his pregnant mother suffered at the hands of his abusive, drug-addicted father.

Virginia rarely becomes attached to these babies. Sometimes she even finds herself wondering why she is working so hard to save them. If they live, they will have to return home. "I think that may be more cruel than letting them die," she says.

She found herself becoming angry on days when Taylor was doing poorly and some other baby, whose parents never visited and didn't seem to care, was doing well. "It's not fair," she would say. "Taylor actually has a life to go home to."

Fran and Carey would bring pizza and cookies to "their nurses"—Virginia on the night shift and Nancy Holt during the day. In return, the nurses guided them through the bewildering maze of Turner, teaching them what was wrong with Taylor and what, if anything, could be done to make it better. Neither Fran nor Carey had been stars in high school biology, but now, like Teresa Knepper and so many other parents before them, they learned everything they could about the problems of a premature baby.

Taylor had a lot of problems, and the root of all of them was the fact that she simply wasn't ready to be born. Most worrisome were her underdeveloped lungs, which, as Sharon Crandell had explained to Fran in the labor room, were far from prepared to take breaths on their own. The ventilator could take breaths for her, but babies Taylor's size are a constant balancing act. Just as one system looks steady and under control, another starts to wobble, diverting attention from the first. The ventilator solves one problem by forcing oxygen in the babies' lungs. But in doing so it damages the lungs and the extent of that damage depends upon the age and strength of the particular baby and the length of time they need to remain on the vent.

As the weeks went on, it became obvious that for Taylor, the damage was severe. She developed bronchopulmonary dysplasia, which Fran and Carey learned to call BPD, a severe scarring of the lung tissue. She also developed something with the deceptively cheerful acronym PIE, for pulmonary interstitial emphysema, which means the tiny air sacs stretch and thin until they become useless. Both of these conditions mean that the ventilator pressure must be turned up if a child is to receive enough oxygen. And each time the pressure was increased on Taylor, so was the damage to her lungs.

Taylor's lung problems, in turn, led to heart problems. The right ventricle of the heart is designed to push blood into the lungs, but scarred and hardened lung tissue makes that job more difficult. Like a stopped sink, the fluid backs up. Eventually Taylor's heart, which was weak and immature in the first place, began to weaken further and fail. When the heart can't pump properly, the strain on the kidneys increases, and they become overloaded and sluggish as well.

Every morning Fran would take a deep breath before entering Turner, not really wanting to know which of these spinning platters was wobbling and threatening to fall. Some days the news was good. During her first weeks of precarious life, Taylor's skin had been tinged yellow from jaundice, meaning her liver was under strain, unable to clear a poisonous waste product called bilirubin. So she was issued a pair of preemie sunshades—actually a square of gauze taped over each eyelid that prompted her parents to joke that she was sunning herself at her private beach. She was then placed under a bank of bright lights, which have been found to lower the levels of bilirubin until the liver can take over. One morning Fran was told that the lights had been removed and that her daughter's liver was thought to be working normally.

Other days the news was devastating. One afternoon the doctors took the new parents into the conference room to explain that a routine ultrasound picture of Taylor's head had found an interventricular hemorrhage, a burst blood vessel in her brain. On the scale used to measure the severity of such bleeds, this one was a 4, the worst there is. Some babies recover fully from these bleeds, Fran and Carey were told, but others suffer permanent brain damage. With Taylor, it was too soon to tell.

Over those weeks, Fran and Carey learned, through books and through their nurses, that there was a chilling side to the deceptively cozy analogy the doctors had used, likening Taylor to a cake that has not had long enough to bake. That comparison implied she could simply be put back in the oven—or modern medicine's best substitute for the oven—and she would come out perfectly done after a proper period of time. But few recipes could handle such interruptions without some unwanted effects, and babies certainly can't. Taylor could face lifelong problems that would follow her long after she left Turner.

Neonatal intensive care units are a product of the 1960s and 1970s. Between 1961 and 1975, only 6 percent of babies weighing less than 1,000 grams, which is 2 pounds, 2 ounces, were able to survive. During the first half of the 1980s, nearly 50 percent survived, a percentage that continues to climb. The success of those units could be seen in the thousands of grateful parents who would have lost their babies had they been born a few years sooner. Success could also be seen in the growing demand for services for these children, who had higher rates of learning disabilities, mental retardation, chronic illness, allergies, nutritional deficits, and hearing and vision problems than children born at full term. No one knew what further complications would surface when these children began to have children.

As they learned more about what was wrong with Taylor, Fran and Carey learned to face the ongoing debate about whether society could really afford to save babies born as early and as critically ill as their daughter. The year Taylor was born, $2.6 billion was spent on neonatal intensive care in the United States, at an average cost of $160,000 per baby. And there were a growing number of doctors and ethicists who questioned whether the outcome purchased by all that money was really worth it. More than 30 percent of babies who weighed less than 1,000 grams at birth would have some sort of handicap that would follow them through life. And those were just the ones who survived. At Hermann, the survival rate of babies Taylor's age and size was 30 percent, much higher than it had been five years earlier, but sobering nonetheless. Of the 70 percent who died, most did so after expensive and exhausting fights to save them. If that money could be used for prenatal care or cancer research, some ethicists argue, wouldn't society as a whole be better off even if these individual families were not?

It is a dilemma that other countries have answered differently than the United States has, at least so far. In Sweden, no care is given to newborns whose prognosis does not look good. In Britain, all babies are given care regardless of their early prognosis, but their status is monitored regularly and if at some point the outcome does not look hopeful, that care is stopped.

Tentatively at first, and then more regularly, Carey and Fran began to talk about how much was too much for Taylor. At first the discussions were not about what they should do, but about how they felt and, more often, how they thought their baby felt. "She must wonder why all these bad things are happening to her," Fran would say. "She must be miserable. How much longer is she going to be miserable?"

One afternoon, when Fran was out of the room, Carey approached Sharon Crandell, who was Taylor's doctor in the neonatal unit, and asked when they should begin thinking of turning off the baby's respirator.

"You'll let us know when we get to that point, Doc?" he said. He is the only parent in memory who called Sharon "Doc."

Her answer was measured and cool. "It would be premature to discuss that at this time," she said. "Your baby does not have a terminal condition. Under Texas law there are requirements for removal of life support, and they don't apply here. I don't think this is an appropriate discussion."

Carey was taken aback. "I didn't say we wanted to do it, I just asked if it's something we should talk about," he said.

"I don't think this is an appropriate discussion at this time," Sharon said again, then moved on to the next isolette.

Fran and Carey don't like Sharon. "Dr. Crandell doesn't give a flying foot about us," is the way Fran puts it. Sharon, in contrast, likes Fran and Carey a great deal, because they are intelligent and eager to learn, if a bit naive. "They're bright enough to ask questions, but they don't always understand the answers," is her thumbnail summary. But she never spent a lot of time communicating warmth and friendliness to Taylor's parents. That is not her way. Instead, she prides herself on being professional and no-nonsense, leaving the pep talks and hand holding to the social workers.

"I know very well that there are any number of people who think that I'm a Snow Queen," she says. "Well, I don't care if people think that I'm a little cool, a little aloof, a little untouchable. You can tell people what they need to know and be nice to them without listening to their life history. If I'm not their favorite person, well, as long as I'm doing a good job, that's fine. There are people who are not going to like me. Guess what? There are just as many people I don't like."

Sharon doesn't look as tough as she talks. She is a tiny woman, with a heart-shaped face, a pointed chin, and thin pale lips. The word that first comes to mind is "pixie." Her voice is equally small and thin, with a pitch like a glass bell. Her clothes are always impeccable, and her earring collection seems endless.

It is a rare day that she doesn't look tired, probably

because she always is. Her official titles are associate professor of pediatrics and program director for the Residency Training Program in Pediatrics. For four months of every year she is the attending neonatologist in Turner, and Taylor was admitted during one of those four months. When she is the attending, she's on call every other night and every other weekend, available by beeper at all hours. She doesn't have to spend all four months in the intensive care unit. If she chose, she could serve a month or two in the special care nurseries, where the more stable babies go, but that is not for Sharon. The reason she likes her job is because of the crash-and-burn pace of critical care.

She is so at home in that world that she doesn't always realize how easily her blunt, straightforward approach is misinterpreted by parents. At times it seems that she is speaking a completely different language from that of the family members she is trying to inform. She thinks that keeping an emotional distance enables her to provide better care. They see only that she's cold and brusque. She considers herself realistic. They think she's unnecessarily harsh. She thinks the baby comes first and that parents should prefer the doctor to spend time with the patient rather than the parents. They see only that she's too busy for them.

Multisyllabic medical talk comes particularly easily to her and she uses scientific terms so automatically she sometimes doesn't notice that she has lost her layman listener. One afternoon, for instance, she was asked by a Hermann obstetrician to meet with a woman who had learned days earlier that her unborn child had spina bifida, a malformation of the spinal cord. On the basis of the sonogram, it looked like a mild case, but it would require surgery within days after the baby was born. The obstetrician thought it would help calm the parents if they took a tour of Turner, where their daughter would be placed before and after her surgery.

Sharon planned carefully for the meeting—she plans carefully for everything—and hoped to use the session to help the family realize that life for this baby could be okay, if not perfectly normal. "The words 'spina bifida' scare people," she said, shortly before the parents arrived. "There are different degrees of impairment, and based on what we know so far, this is a hopeful case."

But she never really communicated that to the tremulous parents. Her words never managed to sound hopeful. She was delivering relatively good news: The baby's spinal lesion was low, which meant that the odds were very good that the baby would have a normal IQ. But the way she phrased it sounded ominous: "She has an eighty percent chance of being above eighty IQ, which is educable."

Her conversations with Fran and Carey were similar exercises in miscommunication. When Carey asked about removing Taylor's respirator, Sharon meant her answer to reassure him and make him realize that it was not time yet, that there was still hope. What Carey heard was, "How Dare You," and "I'm Busy Right Now."

As doctors go, Sharon is more reluctant than many to discontinue life support and is more likely to see hope where others do not. Earlier in the year, for instance, she enraged many of the Turner nurses when she abided by the wishes of a family and kept a doomed preemie alive at all costs for one month. The infant had suffered countless lung collapses and cardiac arrests. The parents refused to make their daughter DNR, and each time her heart stopped, she was resuscitated. Sharon never tried to change the family's mind.

"The nurses' contention was that this baby is continuing an existence where there's no hope of recovery, and the baby is suffering," Sharon said, months after the baby finally died. "Well, the baby wasn't suffering, because she had enough neurologic damage that she couldn't feel anything anyway. It's true that her life was prolonged beyond what it needed or even should have been, but the baby wasn't suffering."

Part of Sharon's approach in that case was based on her fear of the real and ominous realities of the legal minefield of medicine. "Even if I felt strongly that the parents were doing wrong, I was not willing to put my career on the line for that," she says. "I have no interest in spending a couple of years in Huntsville penitentiary on manslaughter charges. I have no interest in having my license revoked. As long as our legal system is as it is, I could never have gone around that family's wishes."

But part of her approach is based on the simpler fact that she hates having to give up. If there are still things that can be done for a baby, she will do them, and in neonatology, more than many other specialties, there is always one extra something that can yet be tried. In that way, Neo, as it is called, is the ultimate evolution of medicine, a measure of the progress between the turn of the century, when children were almost never taken to the doctor, and today, when a preemie can log a $100,000 bill within months.

Neo appeals to Sharon's aggressive, intellectual side. During medical school she had thought of becoming a pediatric oncologist, caring for children with cancer. But her attachment to the patients, one ten-year-old boy in particular, made her decide that she became too enmeshed in that line of work to do it properly. She met the child when she was a student, he died when she was a resident, and, she says, "That bothered me a whole lot more than the preemies even do. I felt like my little brother just died. The babies are easier than the older children. Don't get me wrong. It's not that they're easy, it's not that I don't care about them. But you can't talk to them, they can't talk to you. It's emotionally safer. I need that to do my job and still stay sane."

Fran and Carey didn't really care that Sharon's detachment was her way of providing better care. All they knew was that they needed emotional support that their baby's doctor was not able to give. They felt that she never had enough time to answer their questions and that, when she did take a few moments to talk, she made them feel like potential litigants in the lawsuit she seemed certain they would bring. That feeling was strongest whenever they raised the subject of discontinuing the ventilator, which they did once every few weeks. Each time they asked the question, Sharon would answer in almost exactly the same words, the ones she had learned to use in this era of medical malpractice and governmental rules about the care of tiny children. Then she would write a carefully phrased note in the chart. Most were similar to one she wrote two weeks after Taylor was born, when Fran first found the courage to give her own voice to the concerns that she had gratefully let Carey handle until then: "I spoke with Mrs. Poarch at length about the infant's status," Sharon wrote. "She is concerned about long range care and potential problem of terminal status if infant deteriorates. I discussed with her that infants cannot be discriminated against on the basis of handicap or potential handicap."

Then, as suddenly as Sharon had entered the Poarches' lives, she left it, at least for a while. The attending doctor rotates every month, and one morning when they arrived at Turner, Dr. Eugene Adcock was making rounds in place of Dr. Sharon Crandell. Within days they learned to adore him. In the flow chart of command at Hermann, Gene is Sharon's administrative supervisor in the NICU, and, like Sharon, he has a string of titles that reflect his lack of spare time. Specifically, he is director of the Neonatal/Perinatal Division of the medical school and the head of the Newborn Service at Hermann. He, too, can be a busy, detached man, but he took a particular liking to Fran and Carey, and they spent hours in his office, beneath the wall of baby snapshots, sharing their fears and soaking up his advice. When he delivered news that was particularly good or bad, he would dispense it with a hug, a habit that annoyed many of the nurses, who found it pompous and inappropriate, but which was precisely what Taylor's parents needed.

He played father figure to the exhausted Fran and Carey, a role made easier by the fact that they were only a few years older than his own grown children. He didn't mind their constant questions and demands for answers, and patiently taught them when Taylor's oxygen levels were too low and when her X rays looked worse. With time he worried that they were learning too much, too soon, causing them to panic at minor adjustments in her routine. They were knowledgeable enough to know, for instance, that the goal was to decrease the percentage of oxygen their daughter was receiving from the vent. But they were not knowledgeable enough to know whether an increase of 2 percent in that level was cause for alarm or part of the expected ebb and flow of Taylor's day. He tried to coax them away from the trees and into the forest, concentrating less on the moment-to-moment fluctuations and more on the greater questions, such as whether or not their baby was going to live.

On Gene's watch, Fran held Taylor for the first time.

It was a complicated cuddle. Moving the infant from her warmer meant moving all her tubes as well, and it took nearly ten minutes before the connections were secured and Taylor was wrapped in a sheet of synthetic sheepskin and placed in her mother's arms. Fran sat rigidly on one of the donated rocking chairs, feet flat on the floor to keep it from moving. The fluffy blanket around Taylor gave the illusion of bulk and weight, almost as if she were a regular baby. It took a few minutes, but Fran gradually started to relax. Almost as soon as she did, it was time to put Taylor back again. She couldn't be away from the warmth of her bed for very long.

While Sharon was in charge, Taylor's stay had been relatively smooth, not hopeful, but not alarming either. Gene had held the reins for about a week when the baby began an up-and-down cycle almost as jagged as the tracings on her heart monitor. First, her ventilator failed twice. Between four o'clock and five o'clock one morning the machine simply stopped working. Her oxygen levels dropped dramatically, while her carbon dioxide levels rose, and Virginia ran to her bedside with a hand-operated respirator, which looks something like a fireplace bellows and works much the same way.

Then her kidneys began to fail. It happened when Carey was away on a business trip, the first time he had left town since the twins were born. He had barely arrived at his destination, when he turned around and came back home because Taylor had stopped producing urine, and the toxins that should have been excreted through her kidneys were building up in her body. That can be fatal in the strongest of babies, and Taylor was anything but strong. By the time Carey reached her, she was puffy and even paler than usual. The spot where her feeding line burrowed into her skin was swollen and bright red, and the sight made her father wince. He didn't stay at her side very long because Gene had called a meeting in the peach conference room across the hall, and everyone else was waiting: Fran, Eugene Adcock, Carey's sister, the medical resident in Turner that month, and the nurse caring for Taylor during this shift. Carey gave Fran a quick hug, then held her hand and waited for Gene to tell them whether Taylor would live.

The doctor got right to the point. "You've asked me periodically if you have any decisions to make," he said, referring to the way the Poarches phrased things when they asked whether it was time to consider turning off the vent. "I told you I would tell you when it was time for that. Well, it's time."

He waited a moment for his words to settle in.

"It's been more than three days," he said. "In fifteen years I've never seen a baby recover from a complete renal failure of this severity and this duration. I think the kidney failure coupled with the rest of her problems means whatever we do is simply prolonging the inevitable. I'm very sorry."

He went on to explain Hermann's Supportive Care Protocols, suggesting without saying so directly that Taylor be made Supportive Protocol I, meaning there would be no more trying to wean her from the vent and no attempts to save her with drugs or CPR if she went into cardiac arrest or pulmonary arrest. Fran and Carey had talked about this so often they didn't even have to look at each other before they answered, almost in unison. "That's what we want."

That was on a Friday afternoon. The rest of the weekend was a blur ending with what Fran and Carey believe was a miracle. Without anyone officially authorizing it, the rules of Turner were changed so that Taylor's aunts and uncles could visit, and a parade of relatives began. The stack of stuffed animals at the baby's bed grew so high that the nurses parceled some out to the other patients. Fran and Carey almost never left the floor, holding Taylor as often as they could and taking unsuccessful catnaps on the conference room couch. They made only one trip out of the hospital in three days, to pick out a white dress for the baby to be baptized and buried in, and a second tiny casket, just like the one they bought for Jake, except this one had a pink gingham lining.

In the small hours of Saturday morning, while Fran was trying to sleep, Carey scrubbed his hands and pulled a chair next to Taylor's warmer. He sat there for nearly an hour, with his elbows propped on the rim of the cart and his chin resting on his fists. The nurses came and went, the monitors beeped, and occasionally an alarm rang out, but Carey barely noticed. Six weeks earlier he had gazed down at Jake and said good-bye. Now he looked at Taylor and talked to her, too, but while his soft tone was the same, his message was completely different. He had not urged Jake to fight for his life. He hadn't really known Jake, but he did know Taylor, and he had seen how tough she could be. Although he wasn't at all sure that fighting to keep her alive was the right thing to do, sitting there, watching her ribs throb in and out with each breath, he felt, somehow, that he ought to ask her opinion.

"Do you want to make it, Taylor?" he said. "Do you want to keep going? If you do, you have to hang on. You have to start peeing, do you understand? You have to get those kidneys going. We love you. If you want to stay with us you have to fight back."

By the next morning, Taylor's kidneys had begun to work again. Gene arrived for Sunday morning rounds and had to check for himself after the on-call resident told him the news. "I've never seen anything like it," he said. "There's fifteen years' experience down the toilet right there."

As he was leaving, he stopped to talk to Fran and Carey. Pale and restless, they looked almost as fragile as their daughter. "This storm is over, go home," he told them in the tone he would use on his own four children. "Don't come back here until tomorrow."

They left, but they called the nurses constantly. Each time they called they received news that was guarded but good.

The next morning, the family held another meeting with Gene, where they decided to undo the decisions they had made two days earlier. "Her improvement is dramatic," Gene said. "I would advise going back to the original treatment plan. We'll try to wean her from the respirator and give her maximum nutrition. I would also take her off the Supportive Protocol. If her heart slows, we'll give her the appropriate medications, and we'll do CPR if she arrests."

Fran and Carey didn't say much, they mostly nodded and smiled.

Carey did ask the one pressing question: "Does this mean she'll be able to come home soon?"

"She has a long way to go before she's ready for that," Gene said. "But she's closer than she was yesterday."

Leaving the meeting, Fran realized that she was truly happy, and she was struck by how odd that emotion felt. It had been so long since she'd had a moment of relaxation or optimism that the urge to smile took her by surprise. She practically skipped to Taylor's side and sang a few nursery rhymes to the sleeping girl. When she got home that evening, she folded the white dress, put it in a box in the back of the closet, then firmly closed the door.

The happiness lasted three short days. Near the end of the week Taylor's breathing became labored, and she had several dusky episodes, where her skin turned a frightening bluish gray. Then her kidneys failed again, as suddenly and inexplicably as they had restarted days earlier. The Poarches found themselves back in the conference room. "She isn't going to make it, is she?" Carey asked.

Gene explained in simple language what was happening to Taylor, most of which her parents already knew. Her main problem had always been her lungs, he said. They simply were not developed enough, and they had deteriorated steadily with each week. Babies born as early as Taylor are a bundle of systems, none strong enough to compensate for weakness in any of the others. Her lungs put strain on the heart, her heart put strain on the kidneys, he said, adding that such a linear explanation was accurate but too simple. Nearly everything that happened to Taylor set off several other events. She needed calories to heal, for instance, but the more liquid that was delivered through her feeding tube, the greater the strain on her kidneys. The feeding tube was also a rich site for infection and the antibiotics used to fight the infection could damage her kidneys even further.

"With twenty-five-weekers we're racing against a clock without knowing exactly when the deadline is," he said. "All we know is, if they don't start to do better after a while, they probably won't do better."

"What do we do now?" Carey asked.

"You might consider reinstating what we talked about on Friday, requesting that she not be resuscitated if she should arrest," he said.

When he raised the same issue a week earlier, Gene had presented it as advice and made it clear that it was what he would recommend. This time he presented it as a question, a choice that was theirs, not his, to make. For a moment, Fran wondered why his approach had changed. His next sentence brought her answer, and she didn't like what she heard.

"I want to be sure to say good-bye," he said, explaining that because it was the end of the month, rotations would shift the next day, and he would no longer be the attending physician in Turner.

"I want you to know I'll be available to you if you need to talk," he said. "Dr. Sharon Crandell will return as the attending for the month. She's very good, very smart. She did her training here. I helped to train her."

They did not remind their favorite doctor that they had already met his former pupil.

After a few hugs and farewells, Eugene Adcock left to write a summary note in Taylor's chart. "Day of life 54 with severe BPD and two episodes of oliguria and anuria in past 10–14 days. Success with nutrition has been excellent except for renal failure episodes. Long term survival potential is very uncertain. Dr. Crandell resumes care in the A.M."

Patrick

Patrick once had his picture taken next to his hospital chart. That was several years ago, when he was nine or ten, and already the stack of pages was far taller than he was. He has not grown a lot since then, but his chart certainly has, although nobody has taken a picture recently to compare their relative progress.

The entire fifteen-year-long record does not sit at Patrick's bedside every time he checks into Hermann. There is usually a separate section started with each hospitalization, and the longest of his stays fill as many as a dozen of the pale manila folders. The others are stored throughout the medical center—some on paper, some on microfilm, and some on computer, a chronicle not only of his health but also of the changing technology of keeping charts.

Inanimate and inert, charts nonetheless play an active role in the hospital. In part, they are protection against the future in the age of malpractice lawsuits. The staff uses them to document the fact that risks were explained to and understood by the patient and that a bad outcome was not the writer's fault. Less obvious, but more important to daily activity, they are a method of communication for people who sometimes never see each other but who need to exchange information.

At the end of each shift, one set of doctors and nurses

summarizes eight hours of patient progress for another set of doctors and nurses. When the speech therapist comes to visit, she leaves a note so the physical therapist knows how the patient is progressing. When a pediatrician requests a consult from a psychiatrist, that psychiatrist leaves a note giving his opinion, and the pediatrician writes one back, thanking the psychiatrist for coming. When an order is about to expire, nurses place a reminder in the chart that the doctor cannot easily ignore: a bright fluorescent sticker, in colors that vary with the procedure, that says something like this: "ATTN Doctor. The respiratory therapy orders for this patient will be discontinued in 24 hours. Please re-write specific orders and document need with a progress note."

To an outsider, these charts look like a conspiracy of doctors against patients. Like everything else in medicine, medical charts are a string of abbreviations, and it is not uncommon for the same letters to be used as a code for at least half a dozen unrelated drugs, procedures, or conditions. The only way to decipher these is by context. The letters IVH appear all over Patrick's chart, referring to his intravenous hyperalimentation—in other words, the formula that drips through his central line. Those same letters in Taylor Poarch's chart would stand for an intraventricular hemorrhage, a potentially fatal bleeding in the brain.

At the very beginning of modern medicine, the abbreviations and run-on words *were* a conspiracy of doctors against their patients. Until the mid-nineteenth century, there was little doctors could actually do to cure illness, a fact that was potentially bad for business. For a while, doctors were urged to take the Wizard of Oz approach and hide behind a curtain of omnipotence. A popular manual from 1881, written by D. W. Cathell and called *The Phy-*

sician Himself, is a good example. "By employing the terms ac. phenicum for carbolic acid, secale cornutum for ergot, kalium for potassium, natrum for sodium, chinin for quinia, etc., you will debar the average patient from reading your prescriptions," the book advised, then went on to instruct doctors not to allow patients to become too familiar and friendly because such closeness "has a leveling effect and divests the physician of his proper prestige." In general, Cathell advised, it is a bad idea to do anything that can "detract from your dignity, and lessen you in public esteem by forcing on everybody the conclusion that you are, after all, but an ordinary person."

Books don't officially give doctors that sort of advice anymore, but the abbreviations and internal language remain. Into the twentieth century, as doctors learned how to cure, the complex terms gave specificity that layman's language didn't have. Over the years it took on other purposes as well. It's a shorthand for a profession in a hurry. It's a means of socialization for medical students who use the terms self-consciously at first and gradually forget that "bruise" sounds less ominous to a patient than "contusion" and that most people don't realize that "idiopathic" means "we don't know the cause."

Once you know the language, Patrick's entire life can be found in the cramped, hurried entries in his chart. It begins the day he was born, on July 21, 1972, a few months after his father walked out and a few months before his parents' divorce became final. It continues through his most recent admission to the hospital: the night he arrived in the emergency room shivering with fever and gasping for breath, the decision to put him on a ventilator, the struggle to make him well enough so he would not need the ventilator, the question of whether he should have yet another operation, the meeting of the

Ethics Committee, the debate over whether or not to talk to him about death.

Over the years, there was a dramatic change in the tone of Patrick's chart, and it parallels the dramatic change in Patrick. The early notes are more or less a straightforward chronicle of who-what-where-and-when. There are very few pauses to ask "why." The story told by the chart is that of a big, healthy newborn, weighing nearly 10 pounds at birth, who suddenly began to lose weight. When he was two months old, he started to clench his fists to his belly and scream. Eventually he was diagnosed with Hirschsprung's disease, a fairly uncommon problem, and his would turn out to be an uncommonly severe case. Hirschsprung's occurs when the cells that cause the intestines to contract are missing. Without them, the intestines can't move waste along, and the immediate result is extreme constipation or diarrhea. The trauma this causes to the intestines leads eventually to necrosis, or death of intestinal tissue. Those portions that necrotize must be removed, and Patrick's very first night at Hermann, at age three months, was spent in surgery, where one small section of his colon was cut away. Over the next few years he was operated on nearly half a dozen times. Eventually all but one worthless stretch of his colon was removed and the problem still wasn't solved.

Since he could not digest food through his stomach and intestines, Patrick became dependent on feedings that were given through a tube into his bloodstream. This was a brand-new concept when Patrick was born, and it developed as he did. Until the late 1960s, the only way to feed patients who could not eat was to drip glucose solution through narrow tubes, called peripheral IVs, because they were threaded into the smaller veins that branch throughout the arms and legs. It was an inefficient method, requiring upward of 20 liters of solution a day—the equivalent of eighty glasses of water every twenty-four hours. While the solution was being given, diuretics were used to rid the body of the tidal wave of fluid in the hope that the nutrients would be left behind. Patients did not live long under this regimen, and the life they had was uncomfortable.

During the 1960s, researchers learned to cram more nutrition into less volume. By the end of the decade, they developed more efficient ways of delivering these denser formulas, using larger tubes, called central lines, which were threaded into larger veins, usually where several peripheral veins meet.

Two years of survival was all that could be expected when Patrick first started on total intravenous nutrition during the early 1970s. Month by month he broke that record, to the amazement and curiosity of his doctors. As his chart grew, its tone changed. Patrick was not merely a patient; he was a medical milestone and his case was "written up" in more than one medical journal, bringing prestige to his caretakers.

Periodically doctors tried to wean him from the formula, but that never worked. He lost huge amounts of weight during these weaning periods and, at 56 pounds, there wasn't a lot of weight he could afford to lose.

Patrick always wanted to eat (he particularly liked nachos and pizza), but, as he said to one doctor who promptly noted it in his chart, whatever he ate "quickly comes out the other end." The more he ate the more uncomfortable he became, embarrassed that he would need a diaper in case his body tried to pass food through so quickly that he couldn't reach the toilet in time. "Discussed importance of diapers in cleanliness of bed in regards to infection," one of his nurses wrote on a day when he was particularly unhappy about looking like a baby.

The reason his doctors worked so hard and put him through so much was because they knew that the lines would not work forever. Veins were not meant to handle sharp needles and coarse, irritating liquids indefinitely. They leak or develop hard, calcified clots and begin to collapse. The clots become like huge boulders on a narrow river. Although blood continues to flow by working its way around the clots, the catheter that carries the artificial nutrition cannot twist through the organic obstacle course.

Since they are connected to the unsterile outside world, the lines are also prime targets for infection, and bacteria happily colonize on the plastic tubing. With Patrick, each of these complications reminded doctors of a basic fact of medicine: Despite the mind-boggling progress of recent decades, no man-made replacement is as efficient or as safe as the version nature made. Eating is unquestionably a better method than taking nutrition through the veins.

As Patrick's lines became infected or developed clots, they were removed and other sites were found. Each time this happened his doctors were certain they would never find another usable vein, and the search became steadily more frantic. With each attempt, the lines were placed closer and closer to the boy's heart, the medical equivalent of building a house of cards. Eventually the lines were stitched directly into the heart itself. It was one of those lines that became infected most recently, landing Patrick in the hospital yet again.

For a long time, there was little if any talk of where this constant march to the operating room was leading or when it would stop. No one thought Patrick would live this long, and therefore no one had paused to plan his life. The need for one more operation, one more dose of antibiotics, one more jury-rigged way to keep him alive was accepted without question. No one asked whether the pain of constant infection and surgery was worth being alive. No one asked whether this was medical care or torture. No one asked "why" or "how much longer."

Then, about the time Patrick turned twelve, the tone of his chart changed yet again. Suddenly, everybody who had anything to do with Patrick seemed to be asking all those questions they had never asked before.

In part these new concerns were a sign of the times. Medical ethics became chic in the early 1980s, brought front and center by the case of Nancy Cruzan, the comatose Missouri woman whose family's request that she not be fed through a tube in her stomach was rejected by the state. Medical schools began offering classes in medical ethics. Hospitals began forming ethics committees. Patients, once concerned that doctors would not do enough to keep them alive, now worried that they would do too much. Doctors, at least some doctors, began wondering if part of their job was to let some of their patients die.

All this came as Patrick's health was getting worse. In 1984 he spent almost an entire calendar year in the hospital, and that year forced those who cared for him and about him to see Patrick in a way they had avoided before. What they saw was a boy who was dangerously attached to the hospital.

That is because Patrick has always lived in two worlds. When he was well enough to be there, home was his grandmother's shabby house in one of the poorest parts of Houston. The small, dark living room is the main room of the house, and it constantly smells of cooking. The other rooms—alcoves really—seem to fold into each other so that to get to any place in the house you have to walk through every place else. There is very little privacy for a fifteen-year-old boy.

When he was at his grandmother's house, Patrick would sleep on the spare bed in the single bedroom, where cutouts of eighteen-wheelers are pasted on the wall next to his pillow. At night, surrounded by his gallery of trucks, he liked to close his eyes and pretend he was driving the biggest one as far away from the brown, drab room as he could get.

Patrick's other world was Hermann Hospital. That one is new and clean, filled with familiar faces that lavish him with more than simple affection. When celebrities would visit Hermann, they would stop by to see Patrick, and his chats with everyone from Pat Boone to the Houston Oilers are noted in his scrapbook, as well as in his chart. By the time he was seven, he owned two ten-speed bicycles, both gifts from hospital volunteers. Every Christmas he would make up a list of the presents he expected to receive and distributed it to the amused nurses, doctors, and orderlies. He would get almost everything on the list. His favorite movie changed often, but whatever his choice at the moment, the staff let him stay up well past 2 A.M. to watch it on the hospital VCR. If the floor was quiet, they may even have watched with him. ("Watched *Robocop* with staff this afternoon. No c/o pain during this time.") The morning shift knew not to wake him until 10 A.M., when the playroom opened, because he was simply not a morning person.

Patrick's emotional addiction to Hermann was paralleled by a physical addiction. He had become dependent on a variety of powerful medications over the past fifteen years. "Becoming more demanding with meds," typical nursing note reads. "Wants to know exactly when he can have more and if he sees that you have extra of the drug he asks for the remainder."

He learned what drugs to ask for—morphine for pain, Thorazine to make him sleepy, Phenergan for nausea, diazepam when he is anxious, Tylenol with codeine when his back or stomach aches. These drugs can be given two ways—dripped through his IV line or directly injected, or "pushed," into that line. A "push" reaches the bloodstream much faster than a drip, but hospital policy forbids nurses from giving drugs that way, restricting that practice to doctors. Patrick became savvy enough to page the resident on call—he long ago memorized the number of the page operator—and explain exactly what type of medicine he felt he needed.

Of the two addictions, the staff was more effective in breaking the physical one. He was given placebos often, and about half the time they seemed to make him comfortable. On Javier's instructions, the amount of time between painkillers was lengthened from four hours to five hours and then to six hours. But that plan only worked when he was not seriously ill. With each bout of pneumonia or surgical procedure, the schedule was suspended, and he was given as much morphine as he seemed to need, which was usually more than most other patients would get. Once the emergency passed, the attempts to break his habit would begin all over again.

Weaning Patrick from Hermann was even less successful than weaning him from morphine and codeine. A reward system based on the number of consecutive days he spent out of the hospital only worked for a while. More successful was an open invitation to attend every party on the pediatrics floor, even if he wasn't a patient. That idea came out of Kay's belief that Patrick fell ill before all major holidays, particularly those that involve the giving of gifts.

His most recent hospitalization started just before Easter and dragged on past the Fourth of July. But this one was different from all the others. After two months in the intensive care unit, with a ventilator tube down his throat so he was forced to write rather than speak, Patrick admitted what everyone had long suspected— that he was petrified of being out of the hospital, that he would do anything to be safe inside again, and that he needed Kay and Richard and Hermann so much that he nearly killed himself to be with them.

"Patrick has admitted that he contaminated his line with feces and dirt prior to admission," says one doctor's note. "Says he did not wish to die, just wanted to come back to the hospital."

A psychiatrist who talked with Patrick hours later wrote: "Admits to fouling his own line with feces and dirt and says of his hospitalizations that most he caused himself but some he didn't. He's worried that he may have done too much this time. Doesn't want to die and is afraid of it now."

The chart for this hospitalization is full of death.

From a resident: "Pt [patient] appears anxious. Wrote on paper 'I wish I die' asking for morphine and Valium continually. When asked how he felt about dying, patient stopped writing."

From a nurse: "Patrick wrote me a note stating that he wants to *Die* and underlined Die. I asked 'Do you really mean it?' He then wrote 'Yes, I do.' "

From his psychiatrist, again: "Patrick knows (or seems to know) that he has improved. He now fears going home and the suicide allegations may be manipulations to keep himself in the hospital and under care. He is becoming surlier and more uncooperative."

Finally, starkly and unavoidably, the question had turned to "Why?"

Why put Patrick through further surgery? Why fight to keep him alive when his life had become miserable? Why didn't anyone properly question where all this surgery was leading when it started years ago? If they had projected into the future, would they have done anything differently? What should they do now?

Those who love Patrick were asking the same questions, but arriving at completely different conclusions. To Oria the answer was simple. "I want my baby with me," she said. "I want them to help my baby."

To Richard and Kay it was more complicated, but no less clear. "He's dying in slow motion," Richard said. Don't take him back to the operating room, he said. Don't cut him open and replace the line that he infected stooping down in his backyard, grabbing a handful of dirt and smearing it into the tube that went directly to his heart. If they replace the line again, he will infect the line again, not because he's bad, but because that's the way he is, and he's had enough.

For Javier, both those answers were unacceptable. One moment he was preparing everyone for Patrick's death: "Because of multiple previous surgeries replacement of line would be technically very difficult and hazardous," he wrote in elegant hand with his lacquered fountain pen. "Do not think patient would survive such a hazardous procedure. Would not recommend further surgery."

At the same time, however, he was desperately trying to find a way to keep Patrick alive. He read everything he could find—and there was not much—on full intestinal transplants, which had been attempted on rats in Canada, but never successfully on a human being. For several hours one afternoon he had great hope for the potential of an AV fistula, a man-made tube grafted between an artery and a vein. The central line is put into the tube. Since it is made of synthetic material, it is tougher than a vein, and less likely to collapse. But the surgery department and the infectious disease department nixed the idea. Patrick's system was already so infected, they decided, that the fistula would last no more than three days before it became infected, too.

Javier spoke for hours with a surgeon at neighboring Baylor University, who was experimenting in the laboratory with ways to stimulate bowel cells to grow. He inquired about a new drug being tested at M. D. Anderson that showed some promise of fighting Patrick's rampant infection, and he even raised the possibility of transferring the child across the street so the drug could be tried.

It was Javier's frantic search that led Richard to ask for a meeting of the Ethics Committee. The meeting left Javier feeling no less alone with his responsibility for Patrick's life. The day after the meeting, just after his hasty promise to Oria, he filled two pages of the boy's chart with concern and emotion, baring his pain on the page.

"I have been following Patrick for several years and as his primary physician for the last 7–8 months," he wrote. "His main problems have been enumerated clearly above. I agree that the two main ones are infectious and respiratory. On the infectious problems it's important to point out that he has been receiving amphotericin for over a month at therapeutic doses and that cultures remain positive. In multiple and varied consults with the Infectious Disease team (including at a City Wide I.D. conference) no further recommendations were offered. Specific questions asked were regarding the use of a second drug—felt that it would be too toxic and add very little benefit. How long should he be treated? And there was no specific recommendation. The treatment of choice would be to remove the central line (the presumed source of the infection) but in multiple and repeated occasions in which this issue was discussed with different consultants and experts it was felt that it was not technically feasible.

"This information has been given directly to me. With this in hand we have approached the Ethics Committee who unanimously supported our plans, that is: a) because of the inability to replace or exchange the central line and therefore remove the most likely source of infection which we haven't been able to clear with more than 30 days of Rx doses of ampho, b) his lung disease, c) his renal disease, d) his short gut syndrome, we believe his condition is terminal and will place him on a *DO NOT RESUSCITATE STATUS*. I have discussed this with Patrick's Mom and listened to her questions, and she seems to understand this delicate situation.

"I do not believe at this time we should be too concerned about his morphine addiction.

"Our efforts will be directed toward assuring the best quality of life possible for him given the conditions.

"My intention to talk to Patrick is not to tell him he is DNR but to allow him to tell us where he feels now and to clarify that he does no longer need to put up an act for us."

Eventually Patrick's lungs were strong enough so that he could breathe without the respirator. His infection, though far from cured, was brought under control, and that was more than most people had thought possible two months earlier. There would be no more school for him this year, since summer vacation had already begun, and his wouldn't be much of a vacation anyway since he would have to come to Hermann three times a week for twelve-hour-long infusions of ampho. But as much as he wanted to be brought to the hospital in March, that was how much he wanted to leave in July.

For a short while, it looked as though all the talk of surgery and death had been premature. Javier brought out the exclamation points for his last note before signing the release order: "He will go home tomorrow! He is ready!"

The Hospital

When George Henry Hermann, an eccentric old man with a vast fortune, first envisioned the hospital that would carry his name, Patrick and Armando were, more or less, the type of patients he had in mind.

That Patrick had black skin and Armando was from Mexico might have given him pause. The phalanx of tubes and potions and hardware needed to keep them alive would have utterly puzzled him. But the fact that both patients were poor and had no place else to turn would have fit perfectly the requirements laid out in his last will and testament.

George Hermann was born in Houston on August 6, 1843, precisely at noon. His parents, John and Fannie Hermann, were Swiss immigrants who had moved to the United States five years earlier and opened the first bakery in Houston. He had almost no formal education and entered the Confederate Army, the 26th Texas Cavalry, in 1861, when he was under eighteen. When the war ended and he returned home, he learned that both his parents had died while he was gone. Within two years his two living brothers had also died, and his father's house and a few small land holdings became his.

He clerked in a general store. He drove cattle to market for others, using the skill with horses he learned in the cavalry. Eventually he started to buy and sell cattle for himself, beginning with three calves that he fattened and sold for a $40 profit. He invested the profits from his cattle business in real estate. One day oil was found on some of his land, and he was suddenly in the oil business. The wells on that first tract brought $3,000 a day for several years, an extraordinary sum at the time.

He certainly never acted like one of the wealthiest men in town. He was frugal with his funds, and his daily lunch consisted of a cup of coffee and a doughnut. He never married, saying often that "Wives are too expensive." Nearly all his money was spent buying land.

His one personal indulgence was owning a fine saddle horse, which he rode to appointments all over town wearing his dusty black slouch hat. He became a familiar figure on the often unpaved streets of Houston, a grizzled-looking man, his face all but covered by a handlebar mustache and a graying goatee. Much of Hermann's free time was spent sitting at the bedsides of poor neighbors who were ill, sometimes telling them stories or feeding them soup and sometimes just keeping silent company. When he was in his late sixties, he became one of them, a victim of stomach pains that would turn out to be cancer. He traveled around the country to spas and was operated on more than once at the Johns Hopkins Hospital in Baltimore. At the time, Houston had no hospital of its own.

George Hermann fell ill at a pivotal time in the history of American medicine. Through most of the 1800s, what doctors did was seen as just another trade, like carpentry or farming, that anyone could dabble in if he chose. Diaries of the era refer to doctors who were also grocers, midwives who sewed dresses, surgeons who made wigs. The only methods of cure during these early decades of the nineteenth century were downright disgusting in modern hindsight, and unfortunate necessities even to people of the day. Veins were cut and patients were bled until they fainted and sometimes died. Leeches were used where bleedings failed. Purging and blistering were other preferred ways of chasing poisons out of the body.

If doctors were seen as the lesser of two evils, hospitals were places to be avoided and feared. Though they might allow doctors in their homes, nineteenth-century people went to the hospital only when there was absolutely no place else for them to go. Anyone with any money, sanity, family, or self-respect was cared for at home. Hospitals were filled with the poor and the desperate.

Then, medicine itself began to change. First came the instruments, the first real tools for diagnosing disease: the stethoscope, invented in 1816 and refined throughout the century; the microscope, not even a required subject in medical school in the 1870s but all the rage for attracting patients by the 1900s; the X ray, first used in 1895. These inventions did more than provide a window onto the body; they also gave doctors a new confidence. For centuries, their descriptions of disease were subjective: a little swelling, a lot of fever, a rapid heartbeat. Now they brandished the terms "grams" and "seconds" and "degrees centigrade." It was the beginning of what would become a separate medical language, and doctors then as now were reassured by its specificity and unbothered that it confused outsiders.

This era of instruments overlapped the era of surgery and pain. Nitroglycerin was first taken under the tongue for heart pain in 1877. The patent for aspirin was sold to the Bayer company in 1899. Surgery, which had been done for decades with whiskey or bourbon as the only anesthetic, was transformed during the 1840s when ether and chloroform were first used medically. Able to

survive the pain, patients were soon given a fighting
chance against infection when in 1865 Joseph Lister
(for whom Listerine is named) discovered how to kill
germs.

All of this meant that hospitals began to gain respect.
Gradually they were thought of not as hellholes to
warehouse the poor but places of hope and potential
cure. In 1872 there were 178 hospitals in the United
States. By 1910 there were more than 4,000. Sometime
during those years Hermann began talking to his law-
yers about leaving his fortune to the city of Houston to
build a public hospital. Convinced that the wealthy
would build their own institutions when they felt the
need, he specified in a series of wills that the purpose of
his hospital would be to provide care for the poor.

George Hermann died at St. Agnes Hospital in Baltimore, Maryland, on October 21, 1914, at 1 A.M. Two
days earlier he had undergone surgery for stomach cancer. He was seventy-one years old.

On the day of his funeral, all Houston businesses
were closed by a proclamation from the mayor. Flags
flew at half-staff throughout the city, and the bell at
City Hall tolled seventy-one times. The crowds were
too big for any Houston church, so services were held
at the city auditorium. The procession that brought his
casket there was a mile long and was led by the rider-
less Leo, Hermann's favorite saddle horse.

For days there had been rumors that Hermann
planned to leave his entire estate to the city, and everyone was there to hear the details. The crowd was not
disappointed. The handwritten will bequeathed several
huge plots of land to the city, land that would eventually be used to create several expansive public parks.
He also left $2,619,419 in cash. Of that, a few small be-
quests went to friends and business acquaintances, but

most was intended for the establishment of his precious hospital. The place he envisioned would provide free care to the "indigent, sick, and infirm," the will said.

The will set aside $100,000 to build the hospital and specified that the income from the remainder of the estate be used to maintain the institution. The will also appointed a seven-man board of trustees. Three were named in the will, and the other four were to be appointed by those three.

The philanthropist who made those requests was barely buried at Glenwood Cemetery, near his parents and three brothers, when the alterations of his vision began. In what would become known as the first of the Hermann Hospital scandals, nothing was done about building the hospital for nearly five years. The additional members of the board of trustees were never named. During that time there were periodic accusations that the three men already on the board were simply using their positions to make money for themselves.

A grand jury heard evidence against the trustees, but did not return an indictment. Shortly after the grand jury met, however, the original board members resigned and a new group was appointed by the mayor and the district attorney. The first thing this group did was to change the proposed site for the hospital building. Although he did not specify any location in his will, there is evidence that Hermann had in fact chosen a site downtown, near his family home and accessible to the poor, for whom transportation was a problem. The new trustees decided that location was too small and began construction on the far outskirts of town.

Probably not coincidentally, the new location was near the wealthy white neighborhoods that were being built outside Houston. One nearby subdivision was being developed by one of the hospital's new trustees. A second trustee had close friends and family living relatively close to the substitute site. Though convenient for these men, the location was isolated from most of the city. It was a place so remote that, when the hospital building was finally completed, it had to be ringed with a hurricane fence to keep out the wolves, who were attracted by the odor of the sick and dying.

The trustees also decided that the new hospital should not serve only charity patients. These trustees were businessmen, not healers or philanthropists, and they argued that Hermann's praise over the years of large, prestigious institutions such as Johns Hopkins was evidence of the grand institution he really had in mind. More good could be done, they said, if they built a larger hospital than the one described in the will, one which accepted paying patients in addition to providing free care. They filed a friendly lawsuit in state district court against the City of Houston—the first of many over the next seventy years—asking for the right to alter the will by changing the location of the hospital and increasing the amount allocated for construction sixfold, to $600,000.

In response to objections by the Harris County Medical Society, the trustees argued that they were improving on Hermann's vision. Under their plan, they said, the costs of equipment, overhead, and depreciation could be apportioned between paying patients and charity patients so that more of the earnings of the estate would be left for charity care. The court agreed that the trustees were planning to build an even better hospital than the one Hermann wanted.

The building they opened in 1925, eleven years after Hermann's death, was a palace. It cost $1 million to construct, which was well beyond the bequeathed budget and came largely from investments made with the money in the Hermann estate. It represented the growing hope of medicine at the time and even had its own electrical system, separate from the city's, a necessity because the isolated location meant the hospital could not be hooked to the city's power lines.

The official opening was July 1, 1925, and 35,000 people came to wander the halls during the day-long open house. Those visitors entered through the massive iron gates set in the stone arch at the entrance. They then passed the opened wooden doors, carved then as they are today with winged lions, proclamation scrolls, and cornucopias of fruit. They found themselves in a courtyard ringed with plants and tiled in brightly painted earthenware. In the center was a fountain in the form of a marble cherub, all pudgy cheeks and perfect curls, holding an empty conch shell to his lips as if playfully blowing bubbles. One local paper reflected the mood of the day when it gushed: "Monument to Memory of Pioneer Houstonian Deals Out Mercy to Indigent Sick; Every Cog in Magnificent Machine Functions to Perfection; Mercy Administered to Unfortunates."

In all the articles printed about the new hospital at the time, and there were many, little was said about the actual medical care that was provided at Hermann. Instead, the articles, which ran in publications such as *The Modern Hospital*, talked for pages about the automatic clocks and telephone systems throughout the building, the dumbwaiters and elevators connecting all the floors, and the double doors separating those elevators from the corridors in an effort to eliminate noise. A description of the first patient, Mrs. Sarah Brecheen, explains that she slipped on a banana peel and broke her hip and was assigned Room 208. There is no discussion of what, if anything, was done to repair that hip, but the writer does comment that comfortable bedrest and plenty of sunlight sped her recovery.

There was little discussion of medical cure because there was still little in medicine that could honestly be called a cure. There had been some dramatic gains, such as the development of the diphtheria antitoxin in the early 1890s, and by the 1920s, advances in public health, through vaccinations and common-sense hygiene, had all but stopped the spread of smallpox, yellow fever, hookworm, cholera, and the plague. That was a dramatic start, but it was not a cure, and for a decade after Hermann opened, hospitals were as concerned with their gentility as they were with their science.

Hermann would not even admit patients who suffered from incurable diseases. A list drawn up by the superintendent also forbade entry to anyone suffering from alcoholism and most contagious conditions, such as "erysipelas, diphtheria, measles, glanders, scarlatina, mumps, whooping cough, cerebro-spinal meningitis and scarlet fever." The mentally ill were barred, too.

All that began to change in 1935 when the first sulfa-based drugs were found to work miracles against streptococcal infections and some pneumonias. Until then, a simple swollen, infected finger could require a months-long hospital stay.

For those infections that sulfa drugs could not kill, there was soon penicillin, which was first given to a patient in 1941. During World War II it was reserved mostly for soldiers. When the war ended, it became widely used to treat civilians who might otherwise have died. Countless other forms of antibiotics followed: streptomycin, first used in 1944, which had some effect on tuberculosis; chloramphenicol, 1947, which eventually eliminated typhoid fever; chlortetracycline, 1948, which would be known later simply as tetracycline, and which was effective against bacteria that had developed resistance to penicillin.

Suddenly, everyone wanted to build hospitals. It was during those early miracle years, when the promise of medicine seemed limitless, that the Texas Medical Center began to sprout around Hermann, which had stood practically alone in a forest for its first twenty years. As the 1940s dawned, a multimillionaire cotton trader named Monroe D. Anderson died and left $19 million to the M. D. Anderson Foundation, a heretofore modest organization he set up during his lifetime to provide worthy but unnoticed gifts like the $1,000 it gave to the Junior League Eye Fund to buy eyeglasses for the poor.

Anderson's $19 million legacy created the largest charitable fund in the state at that time, but he left no instructions on how his money was to be used. The trustees of his foundation were searching for an idea when, in 1941, the state legislature granted $500,000 to the University of Texas to open a hospital devoted to cancer research. The Anderson trustees said they would match the state's allocation and also buy the land for the hospital, but only if the proposed institution were built in Houston. The legislature easily agreed, and ground was broken in December 1943 for the M. D. Anderson Hospital for Cancer Research.

That same year, Baylor University College of Medicine began talking of its dissatisfaction with the city of Dallas, where it was based. The Anderson Foundation offered to help the medical school relocate to Houston, granting $1 million for land and construction of a new facility near Hermann and M. D. Anderson. Several months later the Texas School of Dentistry also announced plans to build on the land surrounding Hermann.

In 1945 the Texas Medical Center was officially incorporated, and the Anderson Foundation bought 134 acres of forested land, which it deeded to the new center. The requirement was that institutions built on the land not make a profit but reinvest all money into expanding their surroundings and their services.

One unexpected and lasting effect of Anderson's generosity was to move Hermann Hospital even further from the letter and spirit of its own founder's will. The hospital's commitment to charity care had been shaky from the start and had not improved over the years. Only 100 of the 300 beds in the palatial Hermann building were reserved for poor, nonpaying patients. As the Texas Medical Center grew, the oil and land barons on Hermann's board of trustees viewed the newcomers as competitors and began jockeying to make Hermann bigger and more profitable than any of its neighbors.

In 1947, the board announced plans for a new Hermann building, which would be reserved for paying patients. Two more friendly lawsuits were required to clear the way for this addition, and the trustees successfully argued that they could not afford to provide charity care at current levels without additional income from the new building. The seven-story structure, which would later be named the Robertson Pavilion, opened in 1949, and 4,000 people came to this open house. The building cost $3.5 million, held 395 beds, and was the first major hospital in the country to be fully air-conditioned.

This time around there was significantly more bragging about what the hospital could actually do to cure patients instead of simply making them comfortable. Much attention was paid to the $200,000 X-ray section, which covered a quarter of the first floor and would be one of the largest in the United States. (The old X-ray facilities had occupied two small rooms.) Much was also made about the new diathermy and microthermy machines, methods which have long since fallen into disuse but which were all the rage at the time. And administrators crowed about the modern fever cabinets used to induce fevers of up to 106.8 degrees in patients, the point at which most germs were thought to die.

Their new building completed, the trustees and administrators of Hermann watched the world of medicine continue to change. The death rate in the United States was 841 per 100,000 in 1950, when it began a steady descent that would reach 556 per 100,000 in 1982. Life expectancy in 1950 was 68; by 1982 it was 74.5. The incidence of heart disease decreased by one-third. The number of strokes decreased by one-half. There were 21,000 reported cases of polio in 1952 and in 1979 there were 26.

The tuberculosis wards are now gone, although TB is making a frightening return to most large cities. Young people don't die of infectious disease anymore, or they didn't until AIDS made its chilling appearance. The average general practitioner—and there are fewer of those—now sees a case of rheumatic fever once every eight years. A case of typhoid might enter his office once every sixty years. And diphtheria is so rare, the statistics sound downright silly—one case per GP if his career could span 100 years.

In a way, the easy part was accomplished during the 1950s and 1960s. During those decades, scientists managed to eliminate almost all the ways to die from contagious disease. What remained, what still remains, is more of a challenge: how to stop the body from wearing down or turning against itself and how to correct single parts or entire systems that were faulty from birth or that somehow broke along the way.

The solution has increasingly been to replace or

strengthen those parts, but not really fix them. Like duct tape around a frayed electrical wire, the symptoms can be eliminated but the cord beneath remains damaged. The patched area can work indefinitely but can also spark suddenly, burning everything in the room. So much of medicine is imperfect patching—transplanting organs, breathing through ventilators, cleaning blood through dialysis, feeding through tubes. Even the less extreme examples—insulin shots for diabetes, for instance, and cortisone treatments for severe asthma—are not cures in the way that penicillin and tetracycline are.

In many ways, these changes shaped the growth of the Texas Medical Center. By 1954 there were fourteen buildings where Hermann had previously stood alone. Methodist Hospital had opened in 1951, the same year as the Houston Speech and Hearing Institute. The following year brought what was to become the Shriners Hospital for Crippled Children. Two years later, St. Luke's Hospital was built, as was the Texas Children's Hospital.

Soon the rest of the country began to notice the rapidly expanding complex, and patients traveled from as far away as Canada and Mexico for treatment, much as George Hermann had journeyed to Baltimore. To the frustration of the Hermann trustees, however, theirs was not the institution attracting all the attention. The M. D. Anderson Cancer Center was one of the biggest draws and would eventually become the largest cancer hospital in the country. Methodist Hospital was rapidly becoming a mecca for heart patients, who often arrived without advance notice, sometimes in the middle of the night, hoping to be seen by the medical center's most famous doctor, Michael E. DeBakey. During the early 1950s, the surgeon was one of the best known in the country for heart bypass operations. Much of his fame came from the October 1954 "March for Medicine," when he performed an entire operation on live television.

Eventually, DeBakey had to share his spotlight with Denton Cooley, who came to Methodist as DeBakey's protégé in 1951. It was Cooley who did some of the first open-heart operations using a machine to simulate the work of the heart and lungs. Cooley eventually left Methodist for St. Luke's, where he opened the seven-story Texas Heart Institute, adding yet another building to the Medical Center. It was there, in 1969, that he was the first in the country to use an artificial heart on a patient, while waiting for a human heart to transplant. At about the same time, Hermann's proudest achievement was adding telephones to every patient room and cardiac resuscitation carts to every floor. Its newly opened cardiac care center had a total of four beds. The trustees of the Hermann Hospital estate and the administrators of Hermann Hospital were feeling overshadowed.

It had been more than fifty years since George Hermann died, but surprisingly little had changed about the board of trustees for the Hermann trust. The original members were gone, and their hasty replacements had also retired, but in many ways the men who ran the estate in its modern era were the same as those who had originally been entrusted. They were all men of wealth, power, and prominence who made their fortunes in banking, oil, and real estate. Their political views were not what could be called progressive, and several were vocal critics of allowing blacks into various city institutions.

That the outlook of the board remained similar from one group of trustees to the next was largely because they were linked by friendship and family. Ross S. Sterling, for instance, served on the board from 1918, when he was appointed by the district attorney and the mayor, until 1949, when he died. During those years, he founded the Humble Oil company and served a term as governor of Texas. Upon his death, his son, Walter Gage Sterling, took his place, and became chairman of the board in the early 1960s.

Under the uninterrupted leadership of the Sterling family, the Hermann trustees and those they hired to run the hospital and the actual estate continued the philosophy that hospitals, like oil companies, should strive to be as large and wealthy as possible. When Walter Sterling assumed leadership of the board, the trustees began to look for a major medical school willing to affiliate with Hermann. They believed that by becoming a world-class research facility they would receive the prestige that was being directed at Methodist and Ben Taub.

In January of 1968, the board announced that the University of Texas had agreed to open a medical school in Houston, which would be affiliated with Hermann. In return, the Hermann trustees agreed to a $40 million investment in a new building for the school. It was money the hospital could not easily afford. Its yearly budget at the time was almost $35 million and its yearly deficits were about $7.5 million. The decision was made to mortgage the assets of the estate, which went against the Hermann will. The trustees filed another friendly lawsuit, and the court gave its permission to the affiliation with the University of Texas and to the proposed fund-raising plan.

The transformation to a teaching hospital was designed to revitalize Hermann, but, at least at the start, it had just the opposite effect. The plan seemed to confuse paying patients, who began going elsewhere, a trend that would never really be reversed. In reaction to the flight of the insured, the trustees decided to make further cuts in care to the poor. There was not much to cut. By the 1970s, Hermann's charitable care amounted to only $2.5 million each year. But the board saw even that amount as a threat to the hospital's future, and they announced that all patients who were unable to pay any part of their bills would be sent to the county system. At the time, that meant a choice of Jefferson Davis Hospital, which had 275 beds and was already obsolete when it was completed in 1937, and Ben Taub, which was already too cramped to meet demands when it opened in 1963. Soon Hermann would be sending patients to Ben Taub at a higher rate than any other hospital in the county.

A less public change, but one that would have dramatic ramifications a few years into the future, was the restructuring of Hermann. Many top managers at the hospital, including the chief administrator, were replaced by men who tended to be even more business-oriented and more aggressive than their predecessors. At the same time, several key positions on the staff that administered the Hermann trust were filled by men with similar backgrounds. These permanent staffers are the people who really run Hermann. The trustees set the tone, but the administrators fill in the daily details.

For a while it looked as if the changes in structure would solve Hermann's problems. Layoffs were announced, and services were added specifically to appeal to paying patients. The public relations staff was expanded, and influential politicians were put on the payroll as consultants. Perhaps the most ambitious and effective attempt to change Hermann's image was the LifeFlight helicopter-ambulance program, which was one of the first in the country. It began in 1976 to much fanfare and publicity, and although it certainly served the public good—by 1986, more than 30,000 patients had been brought to the emergency room by helicopter—it was also, not coincidentally, a wellspring of glowing publicity. The Hermann logos were plainly visible from the ground, and at night, Houstonians could hear the choppers flying overhead and think of LifeFlight, because no other helicopter service was likely to be flying in the dark. LifeFlight was called to the scene of nearly every serious car crash and refinery fire, and the nightly news invariably mentioned the victims were "taken to Hermann via LifeFlight."

In 1981, Hermann turned a profit for the first time since the affiliation with the University of Texas was announced. It seemed as if the worst was over, but it would turn out that much worse was still to come. Hermann Hospital was really riding a roller coaster in the dark. It had come up one hill and was poised for a deceptively calm moment before hurtling toward the ground.

The hospital was on the brink of what became known as the second Hermann scandal, and this one nearly destroyed the institution completely. On the first Friday of 1985, a flamboyant, noisy Houston television reporter named Marvin Zindler announced on the evening news that William Bernard Ryan, Jr., a senior vice-president of the Hermann estate, had been charged by the district attorney with stealing $90,000 from the estate between 1983 and 1984.

Zindler is the best-known television reporter in Houston. In fact, polls show he is the best-known *person* in Houston, with a recognition rate of 99 percent, two points ahead of the mayor. His tastes run to white on white suits, white wigs, and bright blue lenses in his glasses. Nearly every time he has plastic surgery—and the times have been many—he announces it on the air.

He is best known as the reporter who broke the story of the Chicken Ranch, a Texas brothel that was immortalized in the Broadway musical *The Best Little Whorehouse in Texas.*

The story he broke in January 1985 will probably never become a musical comedy. Eventually, the amount Ryan was accused of stealing rose to more than a quarter of a million dollars, and that was only a small part of the tangled mess that state and county prosecutors, local reporters like Zindler, and a dogged detective named Clyde Wilson discovered over the next twelve months. What they found was that those who ran Hermann had taken to treating the trust as if they were its owners rather than its protectors.

Although George Hermann's will specifically ordered that all income be used to maintain the hospital, administrators bought thousands of acres of land in rural areas around the county and had hunting lodges and even a man-made lake built so they could better entertain their guests. When they were not hunting and fishing, they were apparently taking gambling trips to Las Vegas with Hermann suppliers and contractors, as well as trips to Europe and Caribbean cruises. Once, several administrators used a plane, leased by Hermann for the purpose of ferrying patients to other hospitals, to fly themselves to the Super Bowl.

Money from the trust was lent to estate officials to landscape their homes or put down payments on new ones. One official wrote himself a check for more than $500,000 in deferred compensation before resigning. Two hospital administrators received bonuses of $44,000 each, and the checks were written ten days after 100 employees were fired for budgetary reasons.

The daily revelations were horrible for employee morale. Christine LeLaurin, who joined the public relations staff at Hermann weeks before the scandal broke, remembers the hardest part of her job was finding copies of the morning newspaper before it sold out throughout the medical center. For several months, those papers were her primary source of information about the hospital she was supposed to represent. "Everyone was stunned," she said of the mood of the hospital staff at the time. "For years the employees were told, 'We're broke,' and were asked to ration their paper clips and use their pencils to the nub. Then they read about hunting lodges and airplane trips. It was enough to make you sick."

There were a handful of criminal prosecutions as a result of the scandal, some jail time was served, and most of the board eventually resigned. Most of the actions that landed the hospital on the city's front pages, however, were not technically illegal. In defense of their stewardship, several of the trustees argued that lavish entertainment and hobnobbing with potential customers is how big corporations do business, and Hermann, from their perspective, was a corporation first, a hospital second, a charity third.

The state of Texas has attempted to change that. Unable to prosecute the excesses of the past, Attorney General Jim Mattox stepped in to dictate Hermann's future. The agreement his office reached with the hospital is a complicated and lengthy one that has kept a state-appointed monitor busy nearly full-time in the years since it was signed. Among other things, it limits the term of office of trustees to ten years, prescribes what sort of investments the board may and may not make, and, most significantly, requires that 10 percent of Hermann's gross revenues be allocated to charity care.

The Agreement, as it is called, is a sensitive subject among people who work at Hermann. Nearly everyone welcomed the chance to close the chapter and get on with the business of taking care of patients. But the knowledge that their employer is vulnerable makes many employees feel vulnerable; the awareness that Hermann is being watched makes them feel that they are being watched, too.

Armando

When Armando's stretcher was wheeled off the LifeFlight helicopter, the machinery of Hermann Hospital went into motion on his behalf. Files were established at Admitting, Medical Records, Billing, and half a dozen other offices. A computer log was started with his name to track his medications, lab tests, and movement through the hospital. A written chart was also begun, and a large white index card was taped to its cover with the message: "If patient expires or if bullet is removed (police need bullet for evidence) call Madisonville Police Department. Speak to Detective Piazza or Chief West."

The chart followed him when he was moved from the emergency room to the Neuro Intensive Care Unit on the second floor of Robertson. He was still attached to a ventilator and still wearing a high, stiff plastic brace around his neck. He was placed at station A, on a rotating bed, a cumbersome setup used for patients who will be flat on their backs for a long period. Sheepskin-covered pads were placed close to his legs and on both sides of each arm. Once the pads were in position, soft-sided leather restraints were used to secure him to the bed so that he wouldn't fall. Three straps went across his body, one each at his chest, stomach, and knees, and two others hooked around his shoulders.

Then, at regular intervals, the bed was rotated from side to side, staying in each position for about a half hour. The purpose of this technological hammock is to keep secretions from building up in the lungs, as often happens with a patient who lies in one position for days at a time. The swinging also causes a patient's weight to shift slightly on the mattress, preventing the skin irritation that could result from constant pressure on any one area.

Lying amid the straps, Armando was scared. During his first forty-eight hours in the unit, it seemed as though everyone talked about him and near him, but never directly to him. One morning two nurses stood within earshot and discussed whether or not he needed to be covered with a blanket, but neither asked his opinion. They decided not to cover him. Had they asked, he would have told them he was feeling chilled.

The isolation and panic were strongest at night. The lights of the ICU never went out, and though it grew quieter, the endless activity never really stopped. He already felt well enough to be bothered by that, and when he managed to doze, he would dream that he was running away from the hospital and the noise. He would awaken suddenly and realize that he still couldn't feel his body. Worst of all were the endless sounds of the ventilator, wheezing constantly at his side. It was like trying to sleep with a large housefly buzzing overhead.

During the day, he could watch television. There was a set mounted to the wall near his bed, and his mother made sure it was switched at all times to a Spanish language station, usually one that played music videos. He loved watching television. He had never had one to himself before. The doctors didn't seem to realize how much he enjoyed this minor luxury, and one day he overheard a staff member expressing pity for him, describing him as "a head on a pillow who'll spend the rest of his life watching that box." At the time he didn't understand what they meant, and not only because his English was so imperfect. He had no intention of spending his life like this, but for the moment it was okay. With all these doctors and all this equipment he was certain that there would be a way to make him better. His mother had promised him that, and he believed her. No one had told him otherwise, which made him certain that the passing doctor was mistaken.

Dr. David MacDougall, the doctor who first examined him at Hermann and was now responsible for Armando's case, certainly didn't tell him. He visited the rotating bed regularly during those first few days. At each visit there wasn't the slightest increase in nerve function, and he became more certain that what he was seeing was not spinal shock or swelling, but total and permanent damage. He shared his growing pessimism with the chart and, to the degree that they would listen, with Armando's family. He decided not to tell Armando until he asked directly. When the patient is ready for the answer, he'll ask the question, David believed. If he's told sooner, he won't accept it.

Norma McNair also didn't tell him. That wasn't the purpose of her visit. As nurse manager of the neurology service, she stopped at Armando's bed during his first day in the ICU, the initial step in forming a plan for his daily long-term nursing needs. He could do absolutely nothing for himself, which meant his nurses had to do everything: suctioning the saliva from his mouth and lungs, giving him enemas, shaving him and bathing him, clipping his nails, brushing his teeth and scratching any itch he might get on his nose. Norma was there to determine what needed to be done and on what schedule it could be done most efficiently.

Mary Coffey didn't tell him his prognosis, either. She didn't feel it was her place. She is an occupational therapist, which is a misleading term, since it sounds nothing at all like what it means. Occupational therapy has to do with the work of everyday life—feeding yourself, tying your shoes, opening the front door. Mary and the other therapists in her department retrain patients to do the things they did without thinking before their accidents. The goal is usually not to do everything exactly the same way as before, but to learn to compensate, using muscles that are still strong in place of ones that are permanently weakened, or using specially designed tools in the absence of sinew and synapse.

Which is why she was confused when she received the consultation request for Armando. She had heard about this patient before she met him—word of a C-1 spinal injury travels quickly in the hospital. Mary had been at Hermann for two years, and she had never worked with a patient with so complete a spinal cord injury. According to the rumors, Armando wasn't expected to live, and he was admitted to the overcrowded trauma service only because he was a candidate to be an organ donor.

"What am I going to do for this guy?" she asked her supervisor when the case was placed on her schedule.

After reading Armando's chart and watching him for a while in the Neuro ICU, she paged David MacDougall. "You wrote this order, so what do you want me to do for him?" she asked him. "We don't usually get referrals on people who are expected to be donors. We'll have to use a lot of our services for him, that's thirty dollars every fifteen minutes. Do you really think it makes sense? Shouldn't we wait until he's less critical?"

David shrugged. He had already thought of the cost

and the potential futility, but he decided to err on the side of hope. "Well, he survived the night," he told Mary, "and we didn't think he could do that, so we're going to treat him day by day."

"What are the restrictions? Are there exercises that will cause more damage?" she asked. "Sorry, but I've never seen a C-1."

"Standard restrictions aren't really relevant here. Do whatever you can. It's not like you're going to dislodge anything. It can't be any worse."

When she finally met Armando, Mary was surprised at how alert he was. When his eyes weren't fixed to the television screen, they constantly scanned the room. She approached his bed, lowered the volume on the TV, and introduced herself. Then she began her standard forty-five-minute initial evaluation. By the time she had finished, he was wearing a brand-new splint on each hand. The devices are made of rubber-coated plastic that fits like a tube around the hand, from below the wrist to below the fingertips, to keep the fingers from curling. Muscles tend to clench when they are paralyzed, and with time they become difficult to pry open, creating perfect sites for infection and dirt. Snapping the splints in place, Mary realized, was a symbol of hope that he would live long enough to need them.

Near the end of he visit, Mary put Armando through the first round of what were designed to be daily exercises. Taking each limb in a firm grasp she moved it slowly, up and down, back and forth, until nearly every joint had been attended to. The constant movement tired Armando, though he didn't feel a thing. He couldn't talk to her during the entire session, but he seemed to welcome the attention. As she left, she wondered what he was thinking while strapped to that bed, but she didn't ask, and she certainly didn't tell him what she thought his future would be like.

Cindy Walker would gladly have told him, but for the first forty-eight hours she assumed he already knew. There are two types of social workers at any hospital—the kind who is quiet and soothing and makes patients feel better, and the kind who is brassy and rough and gets things done. Cindy is the latter. Short and stocky, with trademark red-framed glasses, her desire to do good runs as deep as her Texas accent. Her way of showing this compassion, however, is more often by bucking a patient under the chin than by stroking his hand.

She has been a social worker for eleven years, since she graduated from college with a degree in anthropology and decided that the life of an anthropologist in Peru was too gritty. For most of her career she has marched in and out of the lives of trauma and surgery patients. She likes those specialties because she and the surgeons have a lot in common. "I like aggressive people," she explains. "Surgery's not like medicine where they mess around for days and days. Surgeons decide quickly and act fast."

Cindy's first official act was to sort out the matter of the rotting eggs. Armando's mother is a firm believer in a Mexican folk religion that relies on herb remedies and other rituals that are not standard care at Hermann. The first thing Victoria Dimas did when her son was transferred from the emergency room was to find a supermarket and buy several Grade A Extra large eggs. Putting them in the window near Armando's bed, she believed, would keep him from feeling afraid by warding off the spirits that bring fear. She tucked them near the corner of the windowsill, where they would not get in the way, then recited the Lord's prayer seven times as her own mother had taught her to do. It wasn't long before the eggs developed an odor and the horrified staff threw them away. By the time Cindy arrived, Mrs. Dimas had discovered that her talismans were gone and was sobbing in anguish at the evil spirits that were tormenting her son.

Cindy dispatched that problem fairly quickly, convincing Mrs. Dimas that she could pray with fresh eggs daily and only after the staff placed them in sterile containers. Then she moved on to the next colorful and confusing subject—sorting out Armando's home life. The entire Dimas family gathered in the waiting area by the surgical ICU during Armando's first days there, seeming to increase in number every time Cindy looked. His eleven siblings were there, with their spouses and children, along with numerous aunts, uncles, and cousins, all crying and all staying around the clock, since most had come from hundreds of miles away and had no other place to go.

To simplify things, Cindy tried to ask all her questions of just one person. Logically, that would be the patient's wife. But from the time they were introduced, Cindy found the woman to be nervous and evasive. "I am not clear on the family situation," Cindy wrote in the chart. "Wife referred many questions to her mother-in-law and didn't seem very well informed in general about her husband. They have three children ages ten, eight, and five (the two older ones may be from the wife's previous marriage)."

The confusion stemmed from the fact that Carolyn, fearing that the hospital would frown on her unwed relationship with Armando, had lied and said they were married. It took several days for Cindy to clarify the situation, probably because she never asked directly. Despite all the forced intimacy and nosy questions that characterize daily life in a hospital, sometimes those who work there can be inexplicably shy. By the time Cindy realized that Armando, Jr.'s mother had never married his father, Carolyn had returned to Fort Worth, leaving Armando's life and taking their son with her.

Cindy's basic goal in sifting the family relationships was to see if there was any way that Armando's relatives could eventually take him home, ventilator and all, and care for him with the help of round-the-clock home nurses. It was in Hermann's interest to find some way to discharge a patient such as this, who has no health insurance, and whose care can cost the hospital tens of thousands of dollars a month for the rest of his life.

It quickly became obvious that this would be impossible. A ventilator-dependent quadriplegic is a weighty burden for any family, even the few with limitless funds and free time. This family had neither. There was no room for Armando and his ventilator in the Dimases' cramped five-room house, and there was certainly no room for two full-time nurses. Even if space could be found, the nurses probably couldn't, because workers with the necessary level of training are usually not based in places like Madisonville.

Two of Armando's sisters live in Houston, but Cindy rapidly rejected that option, too. One of those sisters was still in high school, and the other worked all day in a laundromat and came home, exhausted, to care for four children of her own. She had no time, room, or strength left for a helpless, dependent boarder.

Armando's relatives were the first to say they could not possibly take care of him. It pained Mrs. Dimas to tell Cindy that, since she and her husband had always prided themselves on protecting their children. That is why they had fled Mexico for what they hoped would be a better life in the United States and why they worked several dirty, difficult jobs every harvest season. Their life had not worked out at all as they had planned, but they still had their pride. Now they found themselves turning away their son.

"How is he going to return home?" she asked Cindy when the subject was first raised. "We aren't educated enough to run that machine. Something will happen to him, and we won't know what to do. We aren't educated, and it's too late for us to become educated. This is all we are."

Their inability to care for Armando themselves, however, did not keep his relatives from expressing their disapproval over the care he was getting at Hermann. Specifically, they did not agree with David's increasingly unwavering statements that Armando would never walk again. They insisted, regularly and loudly, that if the bullet that they saw on the X ray were removed, their boy would be just fine. The day after he was admitted, Armando was taken briefly to surgery, to have a hole cut in his throat as a permanent entry point for the ventilator tube. When he was brought back from surgery, his mother was confused that the bandages were around his throat and not his head. She had been certain that the operation was to remove the bullet that was temporarily paralyzing her son.

David tried to explain that the real threat to Armando's life would come from surgery to remove the bullet. "The problem isn't the bullet," he said. "It's the damage the bullet did upon entry. To take it out we would have to cut into his brain. He would not be able to survive that operation, particularly not in his current condition."

Unconvinced, Mrs. Dimas asked Cindy for a second opinion "from a different doctor of the brain" and, within hours, yet another specialist stopped by the rotating bed. The consultant's note read: "2nd opinion at family request. GSW neck injury to cervico medullary junction. Bullet anterior to medullary region. Pt will *not* recover. No reason to remove bullet. C spine assessed appropriately. Prognosis for recovery very poor. Unlikely he will be able to breathe on his own. No further recommendations."

When told of the results of the second opinion, Mrs. Dimas insisted that a third doctor, this time from another hospital, examine Armando. The attending physician in the ICU that month responded by asking Cindy to call a meeting of the family, the social workers, the key medical staff, and someone from the hospital chaplain's office. Everyone gathered near the ICU waiting room on Tuesday afternoon, three days after the shooting. The only person missing was Armando, and he hadn't been invited.

There were no social pleasantries to open the meeting. "I think you know everyone here," Cindy said to Mrs. Dimas. When the woman nodded, David took that as his cue to begin. With the help of John Berry, who was the neurosurgeon attending that month, and Alan Tonneson, who was the attending in the Neuro ICU, David explained, once again, what Armando's chances were. This time, he was more forceful and blunt than he had ever been before. For three days he had been tempering his message with hope even when he didn't think there was any. Now he feared that approach had been wrong. He was offering hope as a cushion and a hedge, a way to ease reality onto the family and to protect himself if an odds-defying recovery actually happened. But hope was the only part of the message that this family heard. He would have to speak more clearly.

"We have to make decisions," he concluded, looking

directly at Armando's mother, "and those decisions have to be based on the reality that this is all there will ever be."

Cindy nodded. That's what she had been saying all along.

"Have you talked to him directly?" she asked. "How much of this has sunk in?"

First David and then the others on the case said they hadn't had a real discussion with Armando at all.

"Isn't it time someone talked to him?" Cindy asked, then waited as the question was translated for Mrs. Dimas.

The weathered, weary woman reacted by shaking her head furiously and speaking so quickly that the very adept translator had difficulty keeping pace.

"It's not true, it's not true, you can't tell him that because it's not true. He can walk, he will walk. He can breathe, he will not need that machine. Why do you say otherwise?"

Tears started rolling from her eyes, and she brushed at them with the back of her hand as she told a story she once heard when she still lived in Mexico. A young man, the cousin of a neighbor, was shot, just like Armando. For a time he, too, could not walk, and was wheeled around the town in a rolling chair. But, she said, his family cared for him and his friends prayed for him, and now he can walk. He even has children. She didn't remember his name, she said, but she knows that the story is true. And that was a small, poor village. Hermann is a big modern hospital, she said, as if daring the staff to meet her challenge. Surely all these doctors could cure him. Otherwise she would find someplace else.

There were many people at the meeting who would have been relieved if Mrs. Dimas had taken her son elsewhere. They knew the drain he was about to become on Hermann's shaky resources. But they also knew that there was no other hospital in Houston that would admit him, given his devastating injuries and absence of funds. This meeting, however, was not the place to explain those harsh economic facts. Instead, David slipped a manila envelope from the pile of papers on his lap and removed the X ray of Armando's neck and skull. Pinching one corner between his thumb and index finger he stood up, walked across the room to where Mrs. Dimas sat and held the translucent film up to the ceiling light so she could see the picture.

Even to a layman's eye, it was obvious that nothing in Armando's neck looked the way it should. Near the bottom of the X ray was an area of bone that appeared shattered, like a piece of fine porcelain that had been stepped on. Farther up, where the rounded bulge of skull began, was a small rounded object, stark white and clearly outlined in contrast to the grayer, more uneven shades of the surrounding bone. It was so bright, it seemed to be lighted separately from the rest of the film. Its shape was deceptive, since it had been flattened and fragmented as it hit its target, but there was no question that it was a bullet.

David raised his free hand above his head, then pointed to the spot where his own neck connected to his shoulders. "That bullet entered right about here," he said, jabbing at the area with his index finger. Then he slid his finger upward until he reached the hairline at the base of his own skull. "It stopped here." Running his hand up and down between the two points he explained: "As it traveled it ripped the spinal cord in its path. That cannot regenerate. The spinal cord is what transmits messages from the brain to the body and tells the muscles what to do. The messages can't get through, and that's why he can't move."

By now Mrs. Dimas was sobbing loudly. "Why is the bullet there?" she yelled. "It shouldn't be there. He doesn't want it. I don't want it there. The bullet is why he can't walk. Why is it still there?"

As she listened to the exchange, Cindy found herself becoming annoyed at Mrs. Dimas. The truth was being waved in her face in the black and white of an X ray, and she was refusing to open her eyes and look. Cindy also found herself becoming angry at the doctors and at herself for permitting this standoff to continue. "What do they mean we can't tell him his prognosis?" she thought. "Why are they all so afraid of doing their job?"

Of course she knew the answer. Conversations like the one that would have to be had with Armando are difficult. Debating whether or not to have those conversations was easier. And the discomfort and complexity would not stop with just one conversation; once they told Armando about his future, they would have to ask him certain questions, such as whether he wanted to be made DNR. Stickier still, he might have questions of his own, such as why he was being kept alive at all. He might look at his doctors, who took an oath to cure and comfort, and say, "Let me die." It was a devastating scenario, and it had certainly happened before.

One of the most wrenching cases Cindy ever handled began with a meeting like this one, also in the waiting area outside the SICU. In that case, William Hardy, a sixty-five-year-old man, was completely paralyzed in a car crash. His neck was broken as it smashed against the windshield, and because he had been heavily sedated in the days after the accident, he didn't know of his fate. His three grown daughters and wife of forty-five years planned to keep it that way. They asked his doctors to disconnect his respirator and allow him to die before he could regain consciousness so he would never see what his life had become.

The neurosurgeon in charge of his case, Dr. Hatem Megahed, refused. Dr. Megahed's father is also a doctor and, his son says, "He always told me my job is to try to preserve life all the time. I try to make it simple for myself. I try to save everybody all the time, and I don't mess with these decisions because there are no answers."

Mr. Hardy was alive, he explained to the family, and it was his job as a doctor to keep him alive. If the sedatives and painkillers were discontinued, he said, Mr. Hardy would be capable of making his own decisions, and therefore the family could not be allowed to make such a monumental choice for him. "It's not my job, and it's not your place to decide whether he lives or dies," he said. "I can't turn off a machine on someone who's alive like this. That would be murder."

After a heartbreaking meeting that brought pain but no agreement, the Ethics Committee was called. Cindy still cringes when she thinks of that session. The family accused the staff of torturing the patient. Dr. Megahed chose not to attend, but told Lin clearly beforehand that he thought what the family was suggesting was indefensible homicide. The Ethics Committee met for two hours, then decided that Mr. Hardy had to be awakened and asked his opinion, but once he made a choice, they said, it should be respected. It would be pointless to raise the issue, they said, only to deny his request.

The man's medications were reduced sharply, and that evening the family, the doctors, two social workers, and two psychiatrists gathered at his bedside. Communication was difficult, but through eye blinks and repetition, the psychiatrists were persuaded that their patient understood what he was being told and that he was competent to make a decision based on that understanding. Then they asked the explosive question: Did he want to live like this? Mr. Hardy said no. The question was asked several more times, in slightly different form, and the answer remained the same. Dr. Megahed excused himself from the case, saying he could not bring himself to disconnect the ventilator. Another doctor agreed to do so in his place. The family members said their good-byes, and Mr. Hardy was then given more morphine. When the drug took effect, he was gradually weaned from the respirator until he died a short time later.

The debate within the hospital lasted for weeks. Some, like Dr. Megahed, thought Mr. Hardy should have been given more time to adapt to his life and to re-evaluate such an irreversible decision. Others saw it as a breakthrough for Hermann, a declaration that technology need not be used simply because it's available. The lesson for them was that the patient's right to choose is more important than what the doctor believes the choice should be.

Cindy was one of those who applauded the decision. Medicine has become too powerful, she believes, when it takes away the patient's right to say "enough." She didn't know about Javier's agreement not to tell Patrick he was DNR. If she had, it would have troubled her, but she would also have thought it wasn't comparable with Armando's case or with Mr. Hardy's. Patrick, after all, is a minor who cannot understand a lot of what is happening to him in spite of his demands for information. Mr. Hardy was a grown man who knew what he wanted in life. Armando is twenty-five years old and has at least one child (Cindy still hadn't straightened that out), and he could, with time, comprehend what life as a quadriplegic might mean.

That is why she found herself irritated at the debate over what to tell Armando. *He* was the patient. *He* had a right to know what everyone else at the meeting already knew. There were choices to make, and he was the only one who should be allowed to make them.

David and Mrs. Dimas talked past each other for a few more minutes, and then the meeting broke up, with nothing resolved. Cindy returned to her office, closed her door, and dialed Lin Weeks.

The Committee

After Cindy called Lin, Lin called Randy Gleason, and the three met briefly that same afternoon in Lin's cluttered office. This was an informal meeting of the Ethics Committee, which Lin held every so often when the question seemed simple and no formal request for a full session was made. Cindy didn't want an official meeting as much as she wanted head-clearing advice. She was certain that what she was seeing happen to Armando was wrong. She wanted to know whether someone less involved felt the same.

They each took a cup of coffee from the seemingly bottomless pot in the hallway outside Lin's door, then perched on the metal chairs around her tiny table. Cindy gave a broad outline of the problem. Lin's questions focused on the specifics.

"What exactly do you want to tell him?" she asked.

"How serious this is. That this is permanent," Cindy said, ticking off each point as she spoke by pressing back a finger of one hand with the forefinger of the other. "He's shaky, he's not in good shape, and he'll probably arrest sometime or other. Do we resuscitate him? He couldn't possibly want that. But we can't make him DNR unless he tells us to. He's competent and awake so we have to ask him."

"But the mother won't let us ask him?"

Randy broke in. "*He*'s our patient, his mother isn't. I don't see a problem."

Lin took a sip of coffee and asked, "Speaking of his mother, how many more opinions is she going to get?"

Cindy tried to hold back a smirk. "We're running out of people to consult," she said. "We can't even tell them we'll move him to another hospital. No one else will take him. Even we wouldn't have taken him if we'd known he was this strong. They say he was going to be a donor."

"We don't need the whole committee on this," Randy said, jotting a note to himself as he spoke. "We don't really have a problem. There is no reason *not* to tell him and every reason *to* tell him."

Intrigued, Lin backtracked a step. "He was really supposed to be a donor?"

"Yup," Cindy said. "That's what I heard. We can't afford him. What are we going to do with him? Where are we going to send him? No one's gonna take an uninsured vent-dependent quad. We can't send him back to Mexico. He's all ours."

"What are his chances of surviving this?" Lin asked.

"It's touch and go, but he's come further than anyone thought so far. He's bound to arrest sometime, and if we make him DNR—we'll ask him first, I mean, but he'll probably want it. I sure would."

She paused and then asked the question she had called them about: "We should tell him?"

Lin nodded and Randy spoke: "Someone should tell him."

The next day, Armando was told. At 11 A.M. Cindy entered his room. His mother, Carolyn, and one of his brothers were already there. Norma McNair and the translator followed soon after. Norma did most of the talking as the ventilator wheezed in the background. At one point the alarm on the machine went off, and a nurse came over to check the source of the problem. Norma kept talking while the nurse adjusted the dials.

She told Armando that his condition was permanent. Nothing is 100 percent certain, she said, but we are fairly sure this is the best it will be. She explained how the spinal cord works, how it was damaged, that it doesn't grow back, and cannot be fixed.

Then she described all the things that might happen to him because of the paralysis, further complications that might threaten his life. He would be susceptible to pneumonia because he couldn't cough on his own, and his lungs could clog more easily. If that happened, they would give him antibiotics unless he said he didn't want them. He was susceptible to heart failure because all his muscles were weakened, including the ones that held up his veins and hence his blood pressure. If his heart stopped, they would try to resuscitate him, and she described in detail what that would mean.

When she finished speaking, she asked him a long list of questions, each of which could be answered with either a yes or a no. His answers surprised Cindy.

Do you understand what we're telling you?

Yes.

Do you want to have medicine for infections?

Yes.

Do you want to be resuscitated if your heart stops?

Yes.

Do you understand what that means?

Yes.

You know they will pound on your chest, they may break your ribs, they may use electric shock on your chest?

Yes.

You know you could live just like this for many years?

Yes.

There was annoyance in the blinks now. Armando was wondering when all these questions would stop. He had the feeling that these women wanted him to give up and die, an idea he found confusing since he was sure they would eventually cure him. Mrs. Dimas stood up and put her hand on her son's brow. As she rose, Cindy asked a question of her own.

"You want to live?" she asked, her voice betraying amazement at his decision and admiration for what she considered pure but misguided faith. "You know you can always change your mind about this."

Armando blinked twice.

"This isn't the only time we'll talk about this, so if you change your mind, you'll have a chance to tell us. We'll ask you again."

Norma entered a note in the chart. "Plan is to treat any treatable condition and maximal support as per patient's wishes. He also understands that he may change his mind re: either. Will reiterate these findings again."

As they left the room Cindy whispered, "This guy is gonna survive. Now what do we do?"

The Cost of Care

Hazel Mitchell first learned that Armando was a patient at Hermann several weeks after he arrived, when it was apparent that he was stable and that he might actually survive. Hazel's job is to get uninsured patients out of the hospital as quickly as possible and, until that can be accomplished, to see that their care costs as little as possible.

Armando had been transferred to the intermediate neurological ward nearly two weeks before Hazel came to visit. Intermediate care is just what it sounds, a step less intense than intensive care. When she arrived at his room, he was surrounded by nurses. Hazel didn't stop to talk. Armando barely noticed. From where he sat she was just another stranger with a Hermann ID badge. People with badges and brusque manners were coming in and out of his room all the time.

Back in her office, Hazel pulled out the gray-and-white computer printout of Armando's ever-increasing bill. Every item used at Hermann carries a computer-coded label—every packet of Tylenol, box of rubber gloves, tank of oxygen, tube of skin cream. And every time Armando is given a pill, has the cut on his forehead cleaned, needs a new tank of oxygen or wants lotion rubbed on his dry skin, a nurse peels the labels from the needed items and sticks them into the chart where they make their way through the bureaucracy, into the computer, and onto his final bill.

The charges add up quickly. Each dose of Tylenol costs 70 cents. Swabbing the cut on his forehead costs 80 cents for the dab of hydrogen peroxide, $20 for the newly opened box of sterile rubber gloves, and $2.00 for a sterile sponge. The oxygen runs $5.00 per hour, or $120 a day. A tube of Lubriderm is $5.30.

By the time Hazel sat down to analyze Armando's bill, it had reached $57,020.86. And that was only the first three weeks. Scanning the columns of charges, she realized that some were one-time items, such as the $439.50 for the time he spent in the Hermann emergency room and the $1,248 for the helicopter at a rate of $12 per mile. Other charges would be reduced or eliminated now that he had left the ICU. A bed there is billed at $495 per day, while a room in the intermediate unit is a relative bargain at $410. The Rotorest bed, at a charge of $161 per day, could also be phased out.

Even with those savings, however, the remaining numbers were staggering. The ventilator, hardly a negotiable item, carries a charge of $273 per day. Each time secretions are suctioned from that ventilator, which happens as often as once an hour, it requires a trach care tray: $28.25 each. Every morning his blood must be drawn to test the oxygen and carbon dioxide levels: $93.75. The two pouches of intravenous food that provide all his calories each day: $95 apiece. The saline solution that keeps him hydrated: $12.50 per bag.

These price tags, of course, do not reflect the actual cost of the items to Hermann. A short trip to any local pharmacy will show that no mouthwash costs the $2.30 per gargle that Hermann charges. Each line item on the bill includes a certain amount of overhead. Supplies such as mouthwash each carry a percentage of the salaries of the supply staff, the electricity to light the store-room, and the telephone and mailing costs to order that mouthwash in the first place. Somehow the security officers have to be paid, as do the page operators, the cleaning crew, and administrators such as Lin and Randy. Then a few more cents are added to cover all the patients who never actually pay their bills and insurance companies that reject claims long after services are rendered.

The numbers Hazel cares most about are those that are left when the extras are subtracted, leaving the actual cost to the hospital. To find those numbers she multiplies the amount on the bill by a real-world percentage. The percentages were figured out for her long ago by someone who is paid to do that sort of thing. She carries them with her on a pocket-sized chart.

During his first twenty-one days at Hermann, Armando was billed $13,674 for supplies such as rubber gloves, catheter tubes, enemas, abdominal support binders, foam bed cushions, adhesive tape, and sterile gauze. Hazel multiplied that by .441316 to arrive at the actual cost of $6,034.55. The respiratory therapy bill of $14,076 was multiplied by .374903, meaning it actually cost the hospital $5,277.13 to keep Armando breathing.

The pharmacy bill of $7,940.90 was multiplied by .491065 for an actual cost of $3,899.49. The occupational therapy consultations that Mary Coffey had felt so unfair charging Armando were nearly lost on the endless list. Hazel multiplied the $97 item by .778346, meaning the actual cost was $75.50. In all, the actual cost of Armando's first three weeks at Hermann was $29,837, and there was no reason to believe he would leave anytime soon.

There was a time when Hermann Hospital would not have worried about numbers like these. In fact, there was a time when Hazel's job didn't even exist. She graduated from nursing school in 1967, the era of the Great Society and the first heart transplant. The possibilities of medicine were thought to be endless, as were the funds available to pay for them. The accepted gospel of the time was that nearly everyone with a job was insured. By 1967 both Medicare and Medicaid had been created for everybody else.

"We didn't think about money," said Hazel in a wistful tone she might use to describe a time when she still believed in the tooth fairy. "You thought about curing the problems of the world. Nurses certainly didn't think about money. Maybe if we'd all paid more attention then, we wouldn't all be paying so much attention now."

When Hazel graduated, a patient like Armando probably would have died. Ventilators were relatively new, and portable versions, like the one Hermann was trying to use to send him elsewhere, were not yet invented. There were also no CAT scans, sonograms, test tube fertilization, laser surgery, microscopic surgery, or dozens of other procedures that make miracles but cost money.

It wasn't long before the cost of all that shiny technology began to outpace the programs designed to pay for it. Medical technology is like no other industry, except, perhaps, the military. When automakers design a new car, their flights of imagination are constantly grounded by the question of what the consumer will be willing to pay. But when a surgeon finds a way to simultaneously transplant a heart, a lung, and a kidney, he does not spend time worrying about the bottom line. And once the procedure is available, Americans have come to assume that it will be available to all. Intellectually they realize that society cannot provide a $1 million heart-lung-kidney replacement to everyone. But intellect is irrelevant when the person in need of that replacement is Mom.

Which is why the cost of medical care in the United States was $500 billion, or 11.2 percent of the Gross National Product the year Armando was admitted to Hermann. Twenty years earlier it had been 5.9 percent. The runaway cost of medicine is also why insurance companies began saying "no." The restrictions came slowly at first, but in 1983 the federal government completely overhauled Medicare and Medicaid. A system of Diagnostic Related Groups, or DRGs, was created, essentially dividing all medical procedures into thousands of categories, each with a three- or four-digit code. Patrick's main diagnosis of bacterial pneumonia, for instance, was coded 482.8. His secondary diagnosis, the infection and inflammation of his central line (known to Medicaid as a "Device/graft") was 996.6. His ventilator (Mechan. Resp. Assist. Nec.) was 93.92. When he was given a tracheostomy, the operation was coded as 31.1. When there were complications from that tracheostomy, there was a code for that, too, 997.3.

By the time he was released from the hospital in June, there were fifteen separate categories of problems listed on Patrick's chart. A computer bank both at Hermann and the regional office of Medicaid keeps track of how much the state of Texas will pay for each category. That payment is almost always less than the amount Hermann says it costs them to care for the problem. For many patients, even the allotted costs are never paid. In Texas, Medicaid will pay a maximum of thirty days hospitalization for a patient and will not pay any more until the patient has remained out of the hospital for sixty consecutive days. Patrick exhausted his thirty-day limit by the end of January, for which Medicaid paid $55,835.20. He had not been away from Hermann for the required sixty days since then. His March through June bill was $139,773.96. Hermann absorbed the entire cost.

At least with Medicaid Patrick had some form of insurance. Armando had never held a job that provided medical benefits, and because he had lived in the United States illegally for so many years, he had never applied for Medicaid. He also was not eligible for the Harris County hospital, since he was a resident of Madisonville. Technically, Madison County could be asked to pay his bills, but Hazel knew that the odds of that happening were about as high as the odds of his walking again.

In recent years, Hermann has found itself caring for more patients like Armando who have no way of paying for the treatment they need. Part of the reason is cyclical: to balance the number of uninsured patients, hospitals throughout the country raise the fees charged to insured patients. It is a Robin Hood approach to medical care, with hospitals taking from the insured to give to the uninsured. The insurance companies, in turn, raise their premiums, causing policyholders to cancel their insurance. The result is that 37 million Americans are estimated to carry no form of health insurance, and insurance premiums increased 13.2 percent nationwide in just one year, between 1987 and 1988.

In Texas the situation is aggravated by recent history. The oil bust of the mid-1980s left tens of thousands of Texas workers without jobs and, therefore, without insurance. That hasn't kept those people or their families from becoming sick or needing care. In fact, it means they are less likely to see a private doctor in the early stages of an illness and more likely to arrive at the emergency room when the situation becomes desperate.

Many hospitals can't handle the strain and have simply gone out of business. In 1988, 102 hospitals closed across the country, setting a record for the second year in a row. The greatest number of those closings, nineteen, were in Texas. Nearly seventy-five Texas hospitals, mostly small and mostly rural, closed between 1984 and 1988, leaving more than forty counties with no hospital at all. Others, like Madison County, are hoping to avoid the still growing list. Larger hospitals, like Hermann, have inherited the problems that the smaller hospitals can no longer handle.

As if the state and national trends were not daunting enough, Hermann has a unique set of problems that complicate its attempts to stay solvent. It is a dilemma best described by looking at the hospitals to the immediate left and right. Around the corner, to the east, is Ben Taub General Hospital, the only public hospital in the Medical Center, crammed with patients who meet the county's residency requirements and who do not have health insurance that would enable them to go elsewhere. Well-to-do and insured Houstonians are happy Ben Taub exists, and even happier that they don't have to go there. Lines to see a doctor can last more than a day, except for life-threatening emergencies, in which case the care at Ben Taub is better than almost anyplace else in the Medical Center. Ben Taub is Houston's only trauma center aside from Hermann, treating a steady parade of victims of stabbings and car wrecks.

Standing to the south of Hermann and in stark contrast to Ben Taub is Methodist Hospital, the largest private hospital on earth. The inside of the red granite building looks like the most luxurious of hotels, with antique furniture in the lobby and mauve and blue wallpaper in the airy rooms. Patients who arrive by car rather than ambulance are met by a uniformed valet who handles parking and a bellhop with a red-carpeted cart who handles luggage. All patients can send their clothes out for dry cleaning or ask a barber to come to their rooms. With the permission of the doctor, patients have use of the gym—not a physical therapy unit, but a fancy health club with a sauna, whirlpool, indoor track, treadmills, barbells, weight machines, volleyball nets, basketball hoops, and racquetball courts. Things are even more luxurious on the VIP floor, where patients are served afternoon tea on sterling silver trays.

On the health care spectrum, Hermann is upscale from Ben Taub and downscale from Methodist. Unlike Ben Taub, which gets its money from public taxes, Hermann is a private hospital, operating on revenues from patients, just like Methodist. Unlike Methodist, however, Hermann is governed by George Hermann's will, which requires that a part of the revenues be used for charity patients. Nowadays that means patients with no health insurance who don't meet the residency or income requirement for county care. So the hospital is caught in the middle, lumped by the public with Ben Taub, feeling like a poor relation to Methodist. Hermann redirects its profits—and there haven't been a lot of those lately—back into charity care, while Methodist is freer to decorate its building and hire bellhops. Paying patients would rather go to Methodist, which means even less money for Hermann, which in turn means even fewer of the niceties that might bring the paying patients back.

Though there is only a small side street between Hermann and Methodist, every year it feels more and more like an interstate, particularly to those standing on the Hermann side. Javier Aceves insists he can tell from

a distance which of the medical students in the medical
center library are from Baylor, the private medical
school that is affiliated with Methodist, and which are
from the public University of Texas, which is affiliated
with Hermann and Ben Taub. "At Baylor," he says
dryly, "they dress better."

One day in the pediatric intensive care unit, Kay Tittle wondered aloud how a certain private pediatrician in
town managed to stay in business. "Every patient he
sends here has no money," she said. "How can he keep
going without ever getting paid?"

Another nurse overheard her and set her straight. "He
has patients who can pay, but we don't get them," she
said. "He sends the paying patients down the block. The
question you should be asking is how can *we* keep going without ever getting paid?"

It was a question asked loudly at Hermann that summer. The hospital was already more than $4 million in
debt. The situation would only get worse, and within
the year Hermann would eventually have to close its
emergency room to most trauma patients, meaning that
there would be one trauma center in an area of 3 million people. A victim of a car crash anyplace within the
550 square miles of Harris County would be taken to
Ben Taub. But on the day that Armando entered, that
shutdown was still months away and the hospital was
hoping to solve its problems through stringent cost cutting. The twenty-four-hour cafeteria, often the only
source of food for exhausted on-call residents and families keeping vigils, had its hours cut back sharply, replaced by coffeemakers and vending machines. One
afternoon, just before the Christmas holiday weekend,
dozens of people were laid off, including the entire public relations staff.

During all this belt tightening, Hazel's department,

called Managed Care, did not lose any members. Her role is to plan the release of high-cost and complex patients as soon as they are medically able to leave the hospital, eliminating potential problems that might slow that release.

"Years ago you didn't get that concerned about all this because the patient stayed in the hospital much longer," she says of her job. "In the end he either recovered completely and went home, or else he died. Either way, you didn't have to worry about 'Can he afford his medicines when he leaves here?' 'Does he have someplace to go?' 'Is his house equipped for his new handicap?' But now you do."

As Hazel scans her computer printouts at Hermann, she is an unwilling and self-conscious symbol of something many who work there would prefer not to face: the growing importance of money in decisions about medical care. Is Armando a question of money? Was he really admitted as a donor? If anyone thought he would live, would he have been admitted in the first place?

Medical professionals—doctors, nurses, therapists, even administrators—do not like to think of themselves as businessmen. Many do choose this line of work because the income potential is high, but even they could probably make more money in banking or real estate, and they are drawn to their jobs, at least in part, by the idea that they are doing good. They are not alone in this image of their profession. The public doesn't want to think of doctors as businessmen, either. And they certainly do not want to think that money makes a difference in the type of treatment they receive.

That public fear was first made strikingly clear back in 1960, when Dr. Bedling Scribner invented a small plastic device, the shunt, at the University of Washington in Seattle. The flexible plastic tube made long-term kidney dialysis possible, a development with the potential to save countless lives. Yet the treatment was expensive, and there weren't nearly enough dialysis machines to go around. For the next twelve years, until the federal government began to fund the procedure for anyone who needed it, Dr. Scribner's hospital used a treatment committee to decide who among the equally ill would be given access to the treatment. Those the committee voted against inevitably died.

The decisions were made not on medical grounds, since all the candidates needed dialysis, but on social and economic ones. Who had the type of life most worth saving? Who had the most years left, children to support, the wherewithal to make the most of the gift granted by technology? In 1962, *Life* magazine ran a story about this process, and there was national outrage and shouts of "How dare they?"

Because this very first ethics committee was completely about money, subsequent ethics committees, including Hermann's, have been particularly careful to avoid the subject altogether. Sometimes they can. One brutally hot July afternoon, however, shortly after Hazel Mitchell first met Armando Dimas, the Hermann committee finally had to stop skirting the issue. It faced its first case that was solely and directly about money, and it came in the form of a brown-eyed eighteen-month-old boy named Dexter Advani. The child's parents were originally from India but had lived in the Houston area for several years, where Dexter's father, Mohamad, was an assembly-line worker for a local electronics manufacturer. Theirs was an arranged marriage, and Dexter's mother, Reena, was only sixteen when her son was born.

He was small at birth, just over 5 pounds, and in his first days of life he seemed pale and listless. He didn't eat well either, and the doctors at the private southwest Houston hospital where he was born started looking for a cause. Tests found he had a disturbingly high level of potassium and a low level of sodium in his blood. He was transferred to Hermann and the care of Dr. Susan Conley, a pediatric nephrologist, who specializes in children with kidney disease.

To Dr. Conley, the skewed levels of sodium and potassium meant one of two things. It could be that Dexter's body was not producing a hormone called aldosterone, which helps the kidneys regulate those elements. That would be called hypoaldosteronism, with "hypo-" indicating "not enough." Alternatively, he could be producing the aldosterone but lacking the receptors in his kidney that respond to that hormone. That would be called pseudohypoaldosteronism, with "pseudo-" indicating that "the condition had the same effects as a lack of aldosterone but a different cause." So Dr. Conley did some tests and found that Dexter had the problem with more syllables. He was indeed producing the hormone, but his body had no idea what to do with it.

Of the two, pseudohypoaldosteronism is the harder to treat. The condition is potentially fatal. Potassium helps regulate the electrical system of the body, and too little potassium can cause the heart to stop. Sodium regulates the amount of water inside cells, most significantly the brain. When brain cells are overly hydrated, they swell and press against the skull; when they have too little water, they shrink, tearing the blood vessels on the inside of the skull and causing bleeding in the brain.

Pseudohypoaldosteronism is a rare condition, and the blood test to detect it only came into common use in the early 1980s. It was unknown, except to a few laboratory scientists, when Dr. Conley began her pediatric nephrol-

ogy fellowship in 1975. In fact, the field of pediatric ne-
phrology had been officially recognized by the American Board of Pediatrics as a subspecialty of pediatrics
since 1973, and Dr. Conley was only the 195th person
in the United States certified as competent to practice it.
The relative infancy of the area was one of the reasons
she chose it. New specialties tend to be recognized only
when enough knowledge has developed to make a difference. Had Dexter been born fifteen years earlier, he
would probably have died within weeks.

The job of keeping him alive fell to Dr. Conley, a
cheerful, busy woman whose office wall is decorated
with pictures of children in her care and whose door is
covered with clipped Cathy cartoons. Dr. Conley saw a
lot of Dexter. Born on February 29, he arrived at
Hermann when he was eight days old and stayed until
May 17. His first trip home lasted less than a week, and
he was hospitalized again, for a day, on May 23. His
next trip home was more successful and he was there
for more than two months, but returned to the hospital
August 5 through 7 and again August 15 through 25.
He spent a week at Hermann in September, stayed
home through December, spent two weeks at Hermann
in January, stayed home much of February, spent most
of March in the hospital, was home for more than three
weeks and was readmitted on April 16. He was still
there on July 17, the day the Ethics Committee met to
decide whether he would ever be allowed to come back
again.

In some ways this child was a lot like Patrick. His
life revolved around what he was fed, and three times a
day he was given a carefully prepared formula that was
high in sodium and low in potassium. He didn't always
keep the formula down, however. It was very salty to
the taste and often nauseated him. If he vomited, which

he did often, it would wreak havoc on his entire system. After a while the staff became convinced that he was making himself sick because he liked the attention that resulted. That manipulation reminded everyone of Patrick, too.

In other ways Dexter's life and Patrick's could not be more different. While Oria Dismuke did all she could to remain detached while her son was in the hospital, Mohamad and Reena Advani were constantly involved. Dr. Conley would often arrive in the morning to find them waiting by her office door, ready to complain about rude treatment they had received from one of the nurses in the middle of the night. They were very protective of Dexter, too protective in the opinion of the staff, and at eighteen months he could neither walk nor talk. Dr. Conley was certain he was capable of doing both. "He's smart, and his legs work," she would say, "but the parents carry him everywhere, so how can he learn to walk?"

Whenever Dexter was in the hospital, both of his parents were there, too, which was an indirect reason for this Ethics Committee meeting. His first hospitalization was paid for by Mr. Advani's private health insurance. By the time Dexter reentered the hospital, that insurance had been canceled. Mrs. Advani speaks very little English and was uncomfortable waiting alone with her son, so her husband left work, sometimes for days at a time, to wait with her. He never told his employer why he was gone, believing it was a sign of weakness to share his problems with his boss.

After several weeks a supervisor warned him that all those absences would eventually get him fired and suggested that he quit so he could someday reapply for his old job without the taint of a dismissal on his record. He did. He didn't think about the loss of health insurance. In the United States, he believed, everyone receives all the medical care they need.

Soon each hospital admission escalated into a battle. For a while, convinced that he was still insured, Mr. Advani yelled loudly at the staff in the financial administration office when the computer showed that his policy had lapsed. Eventually Dexter was enrolled in Medicaid, but after his first thirty days, that money stopped because he never spent sixty consecutive days out of the hospital. Medicaid paid $20,000 for the first thirty days of his second admission.

By January, when his unpaid bill was over $100,000, Dr. Conley began receiving phone calls directly from Hermann's financial administration office. In all her years as a doctor she doesn't remember any other calls quite like these. The financial arm of a hospital rarely involves itself directly with the medical arm, for the same reason that the advertising sales staff of a newspaper is supposed to keep its distance from the editorial staff: to avoid even the appearance of a conflict of interest. Such involvement contradicts the universally held truth that medical care is not based on the ability to pay. The very fact that she was being called, Dr. Conley thought, was a sign of how bad Hermann's financial situation had become. The hospital has economic problems, she was told, and bills like Dexter's could break the institution. Isn't there someplace else to send him? she was asked. Isn't there something else we can do?

In April, when the bill was more than $150,000, the Advanis were sent to visit the county hospital, Ben Taub. They did not want to go and refused to bring their son on their first visit, taking only his medical records for the pediatric nephrologists there to read. They planned to meet the doctors first and introduce them to Dexter later.

The meeting did not go well. When the overworked doctor who would oversee the case realized his patient wasn't coming, he took the armload of photocopied records the Advanis had brought, placed them on his overloaded desk, and showed the couple to the door. "Make another appointment and bring the child," he told them. They walked directly to Hermann and vented their outrage on Dr. Conley, vowing they would never walk into Ben Taub again.

Dr. Conley couldn't really blame them. Not because of the ill-fated interview. She thought it comical and presumptuous that the Advanis would screen the director of the Ben Taub pediatric renal department as if they were interviewing prospective nannies for their son, when they were in fact meeting the only person in Houston who was willing to treat the boy. But though her reasons were more complex, Dr. Conley was as concerned as the Advanis about sending Dexter to Ben Taub. She knew from experience and some unofficial telephone calls to friends that most of the frontline care there was in the hands of those with the least experience, the residents and interns. This is true to some extent at every teaching hospital, but at Ben Taub, where much of the senior staff is also on the payroll at some of the private hospitals in the Medical Center, she felt it was particularly critical.

Those interns and residents tend to rotate positions monthly, also standard procedure at teaching hospitals, but worrisome in terms of Dexter. His caretakers at Hermann were constantly amazed at how quickly his condition could deteriorate, and over the months they learned to recognize the early, subtle signs and respond immediately. At Ben Taub, Dr. Conley feared, the lack of staff who knew him well would be life threatening. "They'll have to redo the learning curve over there," was how she explained her concern. "And they won't have to redo it just once, they'll have to redo it every month. We're treating him better and better each time because we've learned to make each episode less serious by catching it in time. Over there they might not catch it and then he's going to die."

She worried about less definable problems, too. It occurred to her that the Advanis were being sent away from Hermann because they had managed to make themselves so disliked in the months since Dexter was born. She personally was exasperated with them. Dexter had an uncle, after whom he was named, who worked as an operating room nurse in an outlying Houston hospital. He would call Dr. Conley regularly, and when she didn't return his call immediately, he would contact the Hermann page operator, say he was Dr. Advani, a cardiovascular surgeon, and ask that Dr. Conley be called to the telephone right away. After a few months, she refused to answer his calls.

Dexter was equally unloved by the staff. "He's a hard kid to get attached to," Dr. Conley would tell the committee. "His parents are there all the time, guarding him, so he doesn't have much to do with any of us. In his mind, we represent the bad things that happen to him. When we walk in the room, he just starts to scream. He's the kind of kid you feel responsible for, but not a warm sort of attachment, not the kind of attachment we get to a lot of our patients."

If Dexter were a more endearing child, she wondered, would there be more outrage at the thought of sending him to Ben Taub? She thought there would be, which is one of the reasons why she called the Ethics Committee.

The other reason, in a roundabout way, was Patrick. Though Dr. Conley was never directly involved in his care, he did have periodic kidney problems, and she certainly knew all about him. As she saw it, Patrick was where Dexter would be in another decade. In the nearly sixteen years that Patrick had been at Hermann, there were countless discussions about his immediate problems but relatively few meetings to plot his future. In 1972 no one asked, "How long can we afford to treat him?" and now the question was moot. Hermann had cared for Patrick for so long that the hospital was now unquestionably responsible for him. But when did they assume that responsibility? At ten years? At five years? At eighteen months? Were they already responsible for Dexter?

Dr. Conley had been to Ethics Committee meetings before, all of them about whether or not to withdraw a ventilator from a hopelessly ill child. She had never been to a meeting about money. She had never heard of a meeting about money. Yet money, she was learning, was the question she would have to answer more often with each year. At a loss about how to answer, she called Lin Weeks, who told Ellen Nuñez to assemble the committee.

The turnout for the meeting was small. The Advanis were invited to attend, but chose not to. Dr. Susan Conley was there, along with another doctor who had been caring for Dexter, but they were the only representatives of the medical staff. The one other guest was Willene Guttenberger, the no-nonsense director of Patient Financial Services. Like Hazel, her job was to keep down the amount Hermann spends on its patients, which often meant finding other places for patients to go. Much of that job pained her, but she firmly believed she worked for the greater good. It would not help anyone if Hermann treated everyone without a thought to cost, then closed its doors because it ran out of funds.

Six committee members were present at the meeting, the number necessary for a quorum. In addition to Lin there were Randy Gleason, the hospital's lawyer, Dr. Jan Van Eys, the head of Pediatrics, Ginny Gremillion, the head of Patient Relations, the Reverend Bob Grigsby, who runs Hermann's pastoral service, and Father Albert Moraczewski, a local pastor.

Dr. Conley reviewed the case and her reasons for calling the meeting. She had the chart in front of her on the table as she spoke, along with a list of the topics she wanted to raise: the relative quality of care at Ben Taub and Hermann; her concern that Dexter was becoming a victim of his parents' poor relationship with the staff and her belief that decisions must be made now rather than a decade from now.

"If he receives the care he needs, what's his prognosis?" Ginny asked.

"He'll never grow out of the disease," she said. "But it seems that once these patients get older, they get a lot more stable. He's always going to have a problem with sodium and potassium intake. But we can find fairly reasonable diets to minimize that. He can take the sodium in pill form several times a day, just put the pills in his pocket and take them as he needs them, which he should be able to learn."

His condition, she said, would be much like a diabetic's, placing restrictions on his diet but not posing a daily threat to his life. Unlike diabetics, his life expectancy was normal—if he made it through those first four or five years.

"Would it help if someone at Hermann talked officially to someone at Ben Taub," Lin asked, "and told them of our concerns? Maybe work out a plan?"

"It would make me feel better," Dr. Conley said, "but I don't know if it will make any difference."

When Dr. Conley finished speaking, Willene Guttenberger began. It was her office that had decided not to readmit Dexter once he was discharged, and she was there to explain why. She reminded the committee what Hermann was—a private hospital that also provided care to people with no place else to go. She emphasized each of the last five words of that sentence.

"We can't take care of all the poor," she said. "If you're eligible for Harris County care, you need to get your care at Harris County. We take care of the others. The goal is to protect our assets and not close our doors. We don't have any deep pockets. There are no deep pockets here."

The committee members had surprisingly few questions, and the two guests left after only twenty minutes. For the next half hour the group mostly discussed whether they should be addressing this case at all.

"I'm not fully comfortable talking about money," Lin said, "but I have a feeling this won't be the last time we do."

"Are we deciding about this one case or are we deciding the future of the hospital?" Ginny asked.

"What difference would it make?"

"I don't know if I'm comfortable making a policy that says it is always right to send people away or it is never right to send them away. I think our role should be deciding each case separately."

As he so often does, Dr. Van Eys clarified the hazy conversation with a single remark:

"It's irrelevant to talk about how we deal only with medicine and ethics and don't deal with money. In this case money *is* medicine. Money *is* ethics. And we are not going to come up with a decision that we think is perfect. We are not a committee of Solomons." He paused, then added, "Solomon's job was easier."

In the end they agreed that society had decided for them by creating a county system for Houston's poor. In effect, they said, being ethical did not require going bankrupt in the process. On the consultation form, Randy phrased the decision like this: "The ethical dilemma is clearly dual—institutional and medical. Institutionally, the hospital must look at the issue of distributive justice—i.e. how much of Hermann's financial charity resources can be expected to be expended on one child? Medically, the ethical issue involved Dr. Conley's in-depth investigation into Harris County's system, where she has been informally told that the majority of this child's care would be delegated to house staff. Should this child be transferred to a medical system in which the attending physician has reason to believe the medical care would not suit his needs?

"The Committee supports the institution's duty, yet agrees that Dr. Conley's concerns be addressed. The Committee offered to assist in the medical dilemma by meeting with representatives from Harris County."

When Randy finished writing, he read the words aloud, and there were nods around the table.

"We agree?" he said.

Nods again but no one spoke. No one signed his or her name, either. Randy gave the sheet to Lin, who handed it to Ellen, who retyped it that afternoon, adding the names of those who were present. The next day, the financial administration office told the Advanis that once Dexter was well enough to be released from Hermann, he would not be allowed to return. Within a week the family decided to take the boy back to India, where he would be treated with a mixture of Western and Eastern methods. Dr. Conley was the intermediary with the airlines, persuading them that her patient was stable enough to travel.

* * *

As she worked her calculator through Armando's chart, Hazel saw no solution in the story of Dexter Advani. Armando does not qualify for Ben Taub, though if he did, she would have none of Dr. Conley's qualms about sending him there. Nor was Armando's family offering to take him home to Mexico. Cases such as his bring to mind an old Chinese proverb: "If you save a life, you are responsible for it." Hermann saved Armando, and now it would have to care for him for as long as he lived.

For now there was little to do besides keeping track of his charges and suggesting ways to save a few pennies here and there. For instance, she noted on the chart, Lubriderm lotion costs about half as much as Nivea lotion. Perhaps the nurses could use more of one and less of the other?

About an hour after she began her initial review, Hazel put her findings into an empty folder, which she marked with Armando's name and patient ID number. She would add to the file weekly despite the odds against any form of reimbursement to Hermann. She approaches cases like this with sardonic optimism. "Who knows," she says. "Maybe he'll win the lottery."

AUGUST

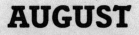

Patrick

Patrick thoroughly enjoyed July. He spent Independence Day at a barbecue at his grandmother's house, and he reigned over his sixteenth birthday party two and a half weeks later. August, on the other hand, was shaping up to be awful. Ever since his release from Hermann at the beginning of the summer, he had been visiting as an outpatient three days each week, during which he was given intravenous infusions of ampho to fight his ever-present fungal infection. In July, the visits were fairly uneventful. In August, they began to border on the disastrous.

Even under the smoothest of conditions, ampho treatments take all day. Often Oria could not get her son to the hospital until 11 A.M., and he would not be released until twelve hours later. The ampho itself requires eight hours to be administered, but there is much more to the procedure than a single drug dripped through his central line. First his system has to be prepared for the side effects of that drug: 480 milligrams of Tylenol in anticipation of the spiking fevers; 16 grams of a thick, gooey drug called Mannitol, which increases urine flow and causes the caustic ampho to pass through the kidneys as quickly as possible, minimizing the inevitable damage; 25 milligrams of Benadryl, to counteract the itching; 25 milligrams of Phenergan to fight the waves of nausea.

As each dose wears off throughout the day, a new dose is given.

With this flimsy medicinal armor in place, the ampho itself could be started. It is not a dramatic procedure. The 32 milligrams of the drug were hung on an IV pole next to his bed in the Pediatric Observation Unit and connected to his central line, exactly the same way his TPN formula was administered to him every night. On good days he would grow bored sitting on the bed and watching television, so he would wheel the IV pole around the pediatrics floor, visiting his friends and eating an occasional slice of pizza or a popsicle from the cafeteria. On bad days he didn't even have the energy to watch television. He would shake with chills as his fever soared as high as 107 degrees, and he often retched and vomited throughout the afternoon. His muscles would ache from his scalp to his toes, and the warm towels and soothing words of the nurses did little to comfort him.

As July became August, the bad days came more often. Not only were the side effects more constant and more intense, but the infusions themselves started taking longer. Javier's fears were coming true. His patient's central line was becoming increasingly clogged, slowing the route of the ampho. Clots had developed along the internal tip, and they were playing host to clumps of bacteria, which happily gather near feeding tubes, drawn by the sugary nutrients that pass through the lines.

First the staff tried to fight the growing blockage with urokinase, the medicinal equivalent of Drano, which was flushed through the line, sometimes for an hour at a time. It was the simplest option available, and when that didn't work, it left only the kind of impossible choices that had become a regular part of Patrick's care.

The next step was to reduce the amount of Mannitol that was given with the ampho, for that drug's thick, syrupy consistency was only making the line blockage worse, keeping him from getting his antibiotics and his nutrition. But without the drug he was left unprotected against the tendency of ampho to eat away at the kidneys. Given the choice, Javier chose to risk the kidney damage.

The flow through the central line improved briefly but soon clogged again, and Patrick's daylong stays stretched overnight two or three times a week. During those admissions, his drugs and his TPN were given to him through peripheral IVs, which are much less efficient than his central line. In a frustrating circle that is the darker side of the miracle of modern medicine, he became weak from the reduced number of calories he was able to absorb and even more vulnerable to the side effects of the ampho.

This left Javier with another imperfect option to consider. A wire could be passed through the central line, like a plumber's snake through a clogged pipe, to scrape out the clots that clung to the tip. The risks of the seemingly simple procedure are twofold. First, the wire could accidentally pierce the central line, making it even more useless. Second, even a successful scattering of the clots could be deadly. The bacteria-laden particles would have to go someplace else, and their route would be Patrick's bloodstream. As they traveled through his body, they would worsen the infection he was already battling so unsuccessfully.

Javier opted for the wire. Patrick received 4 milligrams of morphine and a hug from Richard. Then surgeon Richard Andrassy slipped a thin, bendable piece of surgical wire through the opening of the line and pushed gently, taking care not to allow the wire to reach through the end of the line, which was in the heart. It took two tries before he was satisfied that the line was cleared. Patrick spent the afternoon playing with his best friend, Jason, and nibbling at a plate of nachos. By evening he was too sick to go home. His temperature was 106, probably because of the showers of infected particles that were released from the central line, an unwelcome sign that the procedure had actually worked. The fevers lasted several days, and Javier began to wonder if Patrick would be an outpatient again by the time school began in two weeks. But just as Sally was ready to arrange for a hospital-based tutor, the fevers subsided, almost as suddenly as they had appeared.

"You can get out here," Javier told Patrick, who took a piece of paper and a pencil from the cart next to his bed and began making a wish list of indispensable school supplies.

Taylor

Long after dark, on a sticky August night, Fran and Carey Poarch drove home from Hermann along the deserted Hardy Tollway after visiting all day with Taylor in the neonatal ICU. The road was brand new, a slice of white-gray concrete through the mostly uninhabited woods north of Houston, and few businesses had yet grown up along the route. Often when they made this trip, theirs was the only car in sight for the twenty-mile stretch between their entrance and exit. There were no distractions, no beeping monitors, no hovering nurses, no well-meaning relatives. It was the perfect place to really talk.

When they left Turner that evening, their baby hadn't looked good. A slight improvement in her kidney function had reversed itself, and once again her system had shut down. Her body was so swollen that her skin had begun to stretch and split. Her limbs were stiff, and she rarely moved. It was painful to look at. They could only imagine how it felt.

So it wasn't long before the conversation turned to Taylor's ventilator. This was certainly not the first time they had talked about turning off the machine, but those conversations were about whether they should raise the subject at all. This time, enveloped by darkness and staring at the road rather than at each other, they didn't even question what they should do but talked instead about how to get it done.

"It's just not fair to Taylor," Carey said. "The machines aren't doing anything or helping anyone. And poor Taylor. All those IVs. She's just miserable."

"If it were me in that position I wouldn't want someone to keep me alive by a machine when there was no hope," Fran said. "If that ever happens to me, I'm telling you now, I don't want it."

She looked troubled for a moment, worried that her motives might be misread. "It's not like I'm tired of driving to the hospital every day. I am tired of it, but I would do it for years if I had to. But seeing my baby like that, with tubes and all, what a miserable life.

"Did God mean for her to live this way?"

The question was a rhetorical one that she had asked silently over the past two months but never answered out loud until now. "No," she said. "If she's meant to live, she'll live when they take the ventilator off. If she is meant to die, she will die."

It was time, they decided, to tell the staff what they wanted rather than ask for advice. The car ride crystallized a conviction they had been forming over the past two months: When it was a question of how to cure, correct, or improve, the choices belonged to the medical staff; but when there was no more curing to be done, when improvement was no longer possible, then the choices belonged to the parents. Had they analyzed it, they might have realized that their decision to take control coincided with the reappearance of Sharon Crandell in their lives, a doctor whose choices they so often didn't like. But they would also have concluded that their motives went far deeper than that. The discussion in the car had little to do with Sharon. It had everything to do with an indelible vision of a tiny 3-pound baby in a Plexiglas hospital bed who had never had an unencumbered hug.

Work kept Carey away from the hospital until dusk the next afternoon, and he arrived too late to have his planned talk with Sharon. He and Fran spent that night in the conference room, and while Fran was trying to sleep, Carey tiptoed out and entered Turner in his stocking feet. It was a slow night, and Virginia, their favorite nurse, was sitting in a rocker across from Taylor's warmer. Pointing to the chair next to her, she invited him to sit down.

Carey immediately blurted out the question that he had rehearsed to himself all day. "What can we do to let her die?" he said. The words didn't surprise Virginia, who had been turning them over in her own mind for more than a week, and she answered briefly and without hesitation. "The ventilator can be removed, but only her doctor can decide to do it. You'll have to talk to Dr. Crandell about that."

"Last time I asked, she said it wasn't allowed."

"Situations change. We have done it before."

"Do you think this situation has changed? Do you think I should ask?"

Virginia took a deep breath. This question was harder. The very act of answering, she knew, would overstep the limits of what some doctors thought a nurse's role should be.

"I think she's going to die no matter what," she said. "I shouldn't say that, but you asked me for my personal opinion, and I can't lie to you. I don't think I would have said that to any other family. You know how I feel about Taylor."

They sat silently for a while, staring out the window into the darkness and rocking in unconscious rhythm with the wheezing of Taylor's vent. The few moments of calm were interrupted when two young men wearing green surgical scrubs and a one-day growth of stubble came through the swinging door. They were the pediatrics resident and neonatal fellow who were on call that night, and they were there to check on a newly admitted baby. Their examination took only a few minutes, and Carey followed it from his chair across the room. He understood every word of their medicalese, a grim reminder of how fluent he had become since Taylor was born. When the exam was finished, the doctors came over to say hello to Carey. They didn't know him well, but recognized him from the long hospital nights that were part of all their lives. Carey didn't know them either; after a while all but a few of Taylor's caretakers had begun to blur together for him. But they were doctors, and he knew only a doctor could start him toward the goal he and Fran had set the night before.

"Hi," he said, standing and shaking each man's hand. "I'm glad you came over. I think it's time we talk about removing the ventilator from my baby and letting nature decide."

The question that failed to surprise Virginia a few minutes earlier was completely unexpected by the two doctors. With their backs toward Virginia, they faced Carey and explained that there were only certain circumstances under which a ventilator could be removed. As they spoke, Virginia alternately nodded and shook her head to let Carey know what she thought of what they were saying.

"She's been made DNR before," Carey said, "I think we should do that now."

"That would be possible. You should raise that question with Dr. Crandell tomorrow."

Virginia nodded.

"If you can make her DNR, why can't you remove the machines?"

"If she isn't brain dead, it's against the law."

Virginia shook her head emphatically.

"You're telling me you never remove a ventilator in situations like this, when the outlook is hopeless?"

"I understand that you're upset with her problems in the past few days, we're upset too. . . ."

"Is the outlook hopeless?"

"It's not encouraging, but I'm not sure I would use the word 'hopeless.' "

Virginia shook her head again.

"You've never removed a ventilator from a baby in this condition?"

"It isn't done often."

Virginia's head shook more vigorously.

"What do you suggest I do next?" Carey asked.

"Dr. Crandell will be in first thing tomorrow. Only the attending can make a decision like this."

Carey was afraid that's what the doctors would say. He thanked them, and they left in search of rest. Virginia suggested that he do the same. When Sharon arrived the next morning, Carey was still sleeping, but a note in the chart from the neonatal fellow described the exchange of the night before. Written at 5 A.M., it said: "Father has asked that if his daughter were to arrest that no CPR or code meds be given. He also wants to withdraw support at this time. I told him that we could not withdraw support but we could make her a Protocol I when no CPR would be given and no code drugs. I suggested he speak with the attending tomorrow."

Sharon initialed the note to show she had read it, then continued with her morning rounds.

When he awoke a short while later, Carey did not approach Sharon. Instead, he and Fran walked across the third floor to see Dr. Eugene Adcock, the doctor with whom they felt so comfortable. They sat down beneath the bulletin board filled with baby pictures and told Gene of the decision they had reached and the reaction they had gotten. Then they asked for his help.

"Have you raised this subject with Dr. Crandell since she came back on service this month?"

Carey shook his head.

"So she hasn't said no. Why don't you talk to her?"

"Can she say no?" Fran asked. "Are we allowed to ask for this?"

Briefly, Gene explained the Texas Natural Death Act, one of the more liberal right-to-die laws in the country. It authorizes the removal of artificial life support in cases where the patient's condition is terminal and irreversible and where the machines are simply prolonging the moment of death. Although the law does not require that a patient be either brain dead or in a persistent vegetative state before the machinery can be removed, it is most often applied in those cases, and that, Gene said, might explain the misunderstanding of the night before.

Because Taylor is a baby, he said, Fran and Carey would have to fill out a living will on her behalf. Adult living wills are documents in which patients list the medical treatments they do not want if there comes a time when they cannot speak for themselves. Parents can complete the documents in the name of their children, saying, in Taylor's case, that if she were given the choice, she would not want to live like this.

"Where do we sign?" Carey asked.

"First you talk to Dr. Crandell," Gene said.

"And if she says no?"

"Have you heard of the hospital Ethics Committee?" Gene asked. "It's designed for situations like this, where doctors and families don't see things the same way. I've been to a few of their meetings, and they might be able to help. Let's keep it in mind."

When Fran and Carey returned to Turner, Sharon was still there. They asked for a few moments of her time, and she motioned them to a corner of the nursery. They would have preferred the familiar conference room, where they could sit, but they had the feeling that the doctor was running late, and they opted to forgo comfort for immediacy.

Briefly, they made their case for turning off the machine. Carey worried that his words sounded rehearsed and hollow—after all, he had recited them four times since midnight—but Sharon seemed to understand. She did not, however, agree.

"I wouldn't call the situation hopeless," she said.

"What would you say her chances are?" Carey asked.

"Not good but not impossible. She's still conscious, and she's still fighting. I think we have to give her more time. You don't want to give up on her too soon."

"Aren't we just torturing her?" Fran asked.

"I don't think so. I just don't feel comfortable removing the vent at this time."

Sharon raised the idea of the Ethics Committee just as Carey was about to. "That might be a good idea," she said. "I'm a member, but I've also brought cases of my own." She glanced at the nearest clock. Her days in Turner left her little spare time. "It takes awhile to convene the whole group. I'll ask for a meeting tomorrow morning."

Fran looked alarmed. "It has to be today."

Sharon, in turn, looked puzzled.

"Taylor was born two months ago today," Carey explained. "This is an important day for all of us. We want it to be done today."

Sharon shook her head slowly and glanced at the clock again. "I'm not optimistic," she said.

A few minutes later Fran and Carey were headed back toward Gene's office, which they reached just as he was leaving.

"Can you call the Ethics Committee?" Carey asked.

"Did you speak to Dr. Crandell?"

"She thinks it will take time to get the committee together," Fran explained. "Either it's right or it's not. It should be done, or it shouldn't. We want the meeting today."

Gene called Lin Weeks, explained the case and the fact that it was Taylor's two-month birthday. Lin was familiar with the basic facts; Sharon had already called.

"How about three o'clock this afternoon?" Lin asked.

Fran drove home to get Taylor's white baptism dress and the soft baby blankets she had bought for her twins but never used. Carey walked back to the nursery and sat by Taylor's bed. The nurses heard about the pending meeting and were careful to leave him alone.

He wasn't certain how long he had been there when a social worker appeared and began to ask questions about Taylor. He had never met her before, and he didn't know who called her, but he assumed she was there because of his request to let his daughter die. It was, he believed, the hospital's way of making sure his motives were pure and his decision clear. He was right.

He talked to the stranger briefly, and she was impressed by what she heard. "Spoke with pt's father at bedside today," she wrote in the chart. "He was sitting next to pt stroking her head. He spoke of family's wishes to discontinue support. He said that was not an overnight decision but a long prayerful process. They have considered in the decision the quality of life this child might have and feel that it would be 'no kind of life.' They feel she would be better off in heaven. Their faith in God and belief that the baby will go to heaven with her brother provides comfort to them. They feel their decision will be blessed. Throughout pt's hospitalization the family has visited often. Mr. Poarch talked about all the ups and downs they have been through. Today is the anniversary of the twins' birth and they state today is a 'special day' for them. Mr. Poarch's family are aware of pt's condition and support family in that decision. Father states mom participated in and agrees with decision and will be in this afternoon."

The Committee

Ethics Committee meetings always begin behind schedule, and at 3 P.M., when the consultation about Taylor was set to start, Teresa Knepper was the only committee member seated at the rectangular table in Room 3485. She didn't know that 3 P.M. effectively meant 3:10 or 3:15. This was her first meeting.

Eventually the chairs began to fill, and Teresa relaxed a little. Lin was the first familiar face to walk through the door. The two women had met once, briefly and informally, since Teresa agreed to join the group, and Lin's greeting was warm and welcoming. "I'm glad you're here, we need you," she said.

The other member that Teresa knew was Javier Aceves, her son's doctor, and she was grateful for the company when he took the seat next to hers. A week earlier, five-year-old Matthew sat up by himself for the first time, and as Javier uncapped his fountain pen, Teresa pulled pictures of Matthew's achievement from her purse. Javier was truly interested in the snapshots and asked her to bring them when she came for her next appointment so he could share them with Sally.

The other dozen people in the room were complete strangers. People never introduced themselves at meetings of the committee, so Teresa was left to deduce who was who from the way people spoke and what they had to say. She listened closely as a petite, tired woman gave the history of the case with an air of authority that suggested to Teresa that this was the attending physician and not a mere resident. A few minutes into the presentation, Lin addressed the woman as Sharon, which was as close as Teresa came at the meeting to learning Sharon Crandell's name.

After reviewing Taylor's brief life, Sharon passed two pictures around the table, one an X ray of the baby's lungs and one a sonogram of her brain. Teresa silently compared them to the films she had memorized of Matthew, and she knew right away that these were worse. Matthew had suffered a Grade 2 bleed in his brain, and his pictures had shown a frightening swelling of the fluid-filled pockets known as ventricles. Taylor's bleed was a Grade 4, as bad as these bleeds get, and her sonogram showed patches of lighter tissue, where the cerebrospinal fluid from the ventricles had leaked into the surrounding brain tissue. Like a bursting dam, the pooling fluid ripped much of the tissue in its path. Even after the flood waters recede, the surrounding land remains scarred and damaged.

Similarly, the X rays of Matthew's lungs had shown white blotches, which caused Teresa endless worried nights at the time, but which looked healthy and normal compared with this little girl's. Taylor's lungs were a mass of tiny white circles, like bubble wrap used to protect fragile gifts, and each circle represented a tiny air sac that had stretched beyond the point of usefulness.

As Teresa stared at the pictures, then passed them along to Javier, Sharon continued to speak.

"This baby's chances aren't good," she said, "but I have seen these babies live. When I say I've seen them live, I mean one or two chances in a hundred. But she's one of the ones who could make it. When we talk about discontinuing, it's usually a baby who's clearly dying. With this kid you can't be a hundred percent sure."

She paused for a moment, as if debating whether or not to voice one remaining thought. Taking a deep breath, she continued. "The point is, this baby's brain is still there. Generally we do this with babies who are severely neurologically damaged. I guess I'm a snob. But what I relate to as a person is an intellect. This baby is mentally intact. So it's much harder for me. This is a real baby with a real brain in contrast to someone who's mentally deformed and physically deformed and has no prognosis at all. I don't like giving up."

Across the table, a graying man who had been taking notes while Sharon spoke, cleared his throat. Teresa could read his name, Eugene Adcock, from his ID badge. His title was obscured by a fold of his jacket, but she assumed he was a doctor, and a fairly senior one, because he had no hesitancy about interrupting Sharon.

"May I say something?" he put in. "Sharon is here as the baby's advocate, which is appropriate. I'm here because the parents asked me to be. Lin invited the parents to come, and I suggested they do that, but they didn't feel comfortable, and they asked if I'd come in their place.

"This case centers, as these so often do, on the question of what is futile. No, there's not a one hundred percent certainty that she will die. But it's almost a cliché to say there is nothing in medicine that is one hundred percent. And even if this one is the one in one hundred who makes it, what is her prognosis?"

Sharon answered the question that Gene appeared to mean as rhetorical.

"In my experience, severe lung problems. They're mostly pulmonary cripples."

"Yes. And the parents see that as futile. And I think

it is a reasonable medical decision to agree. We can't save them all, and we shouldn't always try."

"But we're not supposed to be deciding based on the quality of life," Sharon said.

"In this case that's part of the equation."

The silence that followed gave Teresa the feeling that the meeting was winding to a close, and she realized that within minutes she would be asked to vote on the future of this baby she had never seen. She wasn't ready to do that. She still had too many questions.

The idea of asking those questions, however, intimidated her. In fact, everything about this committee intimidated her. The group back in Florida had been easier for her to face. It was smaller, only half a dozen people, and the members had become ethicists together, sharing reading material and debating philosophical points. They accepted her lack of medical training and were eager to help her learn.

At Hermann, she sensed she was playing in a bigger league. They all seemed perfectly nice, but they also seemed busier and more aloof. There would be no helping hands here. Yet Lin had told her to be herself and to speak up when she had something to say. She would only be of use to the committee and the patients whose cases were being heard if she joined in. So she did.

"Are the parents basing this decision on the fact that their baby may die, or on the way they think her life will be if she lives?" she said.

Gene looked at her quizzically. Sharon tilted her head and glanced toward Lin with an expression that asked, "Who *is* this woman?"

Teresa continued in a shaky voice. "I'm asking this because the future can seem awful at first," she said, "and they might think they can't deal with her if she

survives. But once the first shock is over and they have
time to get used to her, they might feel differently."

Teresa was thinking, as usual, of Matthew. In the
days after he was born, she was constantly afraid that
he would die but equally petrified that he would live.
Over the years she has stopped pitying him, because he
spends so little time pitying himself. The way she describes it, her son doesn't think of his life as lacking. In
fact, he thinks the kids without wheelchairs and without
cerebral palsy are the ones who are different. If an able-
bodied healthy person were suddenly trapped in her
son's world, she realizes, he would feel imprisoned and
worthless. But Matthew has never known another way,
and because he doesn't realize what he has lost, he
doesn't mourn.

"Just because this life isn't what the parents would
want or you or I would want," she said, "does that
mean the baby wouldn't want it?"

Though hardly intended that way, there was perhaps
no other question that could have made the committee
more uncomfortable. It was one of the few pure, basic
questions of medical ethics, and one to which they had
no answer. By asking about one specific baby, Teresa
had cut to the heart of the zigzagging history of ethics
committees in general. The question she asked is the
reason why these committees have become fixtures in
most hospitals. It has no answer, yet it is answered every day.

Fifteen years after the establishment of the first dialysis allocation ethics committee in Washington State,
came the second ethics committee, ordered into existence by a New Jersey court. In 1975, Karen Ann
Quinlan lapsed into a coma. Three months later her parents asked her doctors to disconnect her respirator.
When the doctors refused, the parents took their pleas

to the New Jersey Supreme Court, which required that the Quinlans meet with a group of doctors and ethicists. If the group determined there was no chance Karen would recover, the court said, her life-support systems could be removed "without criminal or civil liability" to anyone involved in the decision.

The Quinlan committee was not really an ethics committee, since it ruled only on the probable outcome of the case rather than the murkier realms of morality and humanity. Those questions would not become full-scale committee fodder for another decade, in response to the painful lives of the so-called Doe babies. In 1982, in Bloomington, Indiana, the first of these babies was born with Down's syndrome and an incomplete esophagus. All but one of the family's doctors recommended surgery to connect the esophagus to the stomach; without such surgery the baby, known as Baby Doe, could not live. One doctor vehemently disagreed, saying that the severity of the baby's birth defects would mean a life not worth living. The boy's parent decided to withhold surgery, and the Indiana Supreme Court upheld their decision.

A year after Baby Doe died, a baby known publicly only as Keri-Lyn was born in a Long Island hospital. She had spina bifida, an incomplete closure of the spinal column, which leaves the spinal cord and nerves exposed. Though surgery might allow her to live for twenty years, her parents refused to give permission for the operation, a decision supported by most of the baby's doctors. But A. Lawrence Washburn, an antiabortion activist, heard of the case, and insisted that a court require the operation over the objections of the parents. Eventually the U.S. Justice Department became involved in the case, which was known as Baby Jane Doe.

The courts upheld the parents' decision (and the child's spine closed on its own). The two Baby Doe cases, however, had ramifications that went beyond their individual outcomes. They bracketed the creation of the so-called Baby Doe Regs—federal regulations which, at first, effectively made it a crime to withhold care from any handicapped infant, meaning that doctors would have to do absolutely everything for every handicapped baby, regardless of the prognosis. That brought a howl of protest from doctors and hospitals nationwide, and the rules were softened so that the responsibility for protecting those newborns was put back into the hands of a hospital committee. The ethics committee had arrived.

But what had it arrived to? The Quinlan committee and the Baby Doe committee were each formed for what were essentially contradictory reasons. The Baby Doe Regs were based on the premise that the patient needed to be defended from doctors and family members. The Quinlan committee was based on the opposite premise, that doctors and family members needed shelter in numbers from the courts and the reassurance that they were doing the right thing. Each approach would inspire a different answer to Teresa's question: "Are the parents basing this decision on the fact that their baby may die, or on the way they think her life will be if she lives?" No wonder there was silence.

It was Gene Adcock who answered her, not with a sweeping statement that covered all ethical dilemmas, but with a specific opinion about what felt right to him in this particular case. "I think there are some lives that aren't really lives," he said, "but I don't think that is the question here. I think these parents see what this baby is going through now, and they know that all the suffering isn't doing anything but prolonging her death, and they want to stop that suffering."

Teresa nodded. It was an answer she could live with. If Matthew had been in this same situation, it would have been the decision she would have wanted for him.

Lin interrupted with a change of subject. "Are you sure the parents won't come in?" she asked Gene. "I think it might be helpful for them later on. When they look back, it might help them to have the memory of a dozen professionals saying, 'Yes, we agree, this is the right thing.' "

"They're sure it's the right thing," Gene said. "They see this meeting as a hospital protocol, not something designed to help them."

"I know they're angry," Lin answered. "They see this as a bunch of bureaucrats with their red tape trying to stop them because first one attending says, 'Okay' and then, when they're ready to take that advice, another one says, 'No, stop.' "

"If you think they should be here, I could ask them again," Gene volunteered, then he stood up and walked toward the door. Sharon followed. After all, this was still her case.

As the door clicked closed behind them, a buzz of conversation began among the members who remained in the room, much the way many cocktail parties come alive when the object of juicy gossip finally leaves. Almost none of the talk was about the baby or her parents, Teresa noticed; almost all of it was about Sharon Crandell.

"It's not the family who needed help here, it's Sharon."

"Are we really supposed to be here to hold hands with doctors who can't bear to do their jobs?"

"I think she's just worried about being sued."

"We spent $300,000 and turned away multiple trans-
fers, and the outcome was the same. It never should
have gotten this far."

Even Teresa found herself discussing the doctor to
whom she had not yet been officially introduced.

"I hope she doesn't cry in front of the parents," she
said. "It may make them wonder if they're really doing
the right thing."

Randy Gleason did not join the conversation, but sat
huddled over the yellow and white consultation form,
scribbling what he took to be the consensus of the committee. When he finished, he rapped the table for silence, then read his handiwork to the group: "The
opinion of the Institutional Ethics Committee is that the
patient has a terminal condition and that extraordinary
measures are merely prolonging the moment of death.
Consistent with the wishes of the parents, and the medical opinion of the treating physicians, it would be appropriate to withdraw all extraordinary medical
measures including mechanical ventilatory supports. As
always, comfort measures should be maintained with
special consideration to the dying process after termina-
tion of extraordinary support."

When there was no objection from any corner of
the table, Randy placed an "X" in the box labeled
"unanimous" and wrote in the names of the members
who had attended the meeting: Steve Allen, Javier
Aceves, Lynn Walts, Father Moraczewski, Ginny
Gremillion, and Teresa Knepper. Before he entered
Teresa's name, he had to ask her how to spell it. As
he finished writing, Sharon and Gene returned without Fran and Carey.

"They say any decision should be based on the facts,
not on their emotions or how you feel about them,"
Gene explained.

Randy handed Sharon a copy of the opinion so she could file it in Taylor's chart, which was still labeled "Poarch Girl A."

"Are you going to be okay?" he asked quietly, with his back to the rest of the group.

"I can do it," Sharon said, shrugging one shoulder and lifting her hand to wipe a single tear. "It's hard for me to take any baby off a ventilator, which is why I came to the committee, for moral support. I need to have someone who's not emotionally involved to say, 'Yes, this is a rational request.' "

"You've got that," Randy said. "Let me know if I can help."

It was Gene who told Fran and Carey about the outcome of the meeting. He found them where they had been all afternoon, in the conference room across from Turner, with their parents. After explaining that the decision had been unanimous, he asked them what he could do to make their daughter's death easier for them to bear. Did they want a chaplain present? Did they have any questions they wanted to ask?

"Don't make it easier for us, make it easier for her," Carey said.

"I want to be with her," Fran said, "so I can hold her hand."

Gently and carefully Gene explained what would be done for Taylor, the legal papers that would have to be signed before the machine was removed, the drugs she would be given so she would feel no pain, the way she might look as she died. Fran nodded as he spoke, but she really didn't hear a word. She felt surrounded by a dense fog, like an airplane in a cloud, aware that people she loved were nearby but unable to reach them. Her head felt heavy, her chest felt even heavier, and she feared that if she tried to stand she would collapse from the physical weight of her emotions. So she sat and nodded, hoping that Carey was really listening and could make the decisions for her.

When there was nothing left to say, the new parents left their parents and walked across the hall to the nursery. Sharon was at Taylor's bedside, and she looked as if she had been crying. Fran and Carey stared down at the baby and began crying, too. Theirs were steady, matter-of-fact tears, and they didn't even reach to stop them as they fell because that would have taken energy that they didn't have.

Gene picked up Taylor's chart and turned to the first available page. "5:30 P.M.," he wrote. "This patient is well known to me over 35+ days. I agree she is terminally ill and further therapy is futile."

He handed the notebook to Sharon who wrote a note of her own: "Infant with stage IV, severe BPD, renal failure, grace IV IVH without PHH, infant is terminally ill and intensive therapy will not alter her inevitable course. The parents have requested withdrawal of ventilatory support. That request has been supported by the institutional ethics committee."

Then it was Fran and Carey's turn. Following Randy's precise instructions, Sharon wrote a paragraph for Taylor's parents to sign. "On behalf of our daughter Taylor Poarch, under the Texas Natural Death Act, we have requested withdrawal of ventilatory support. We understand that her condition is terminal and that further life-sustaining procedures would only serve to prolong her death." Carey signed first in shaky hand. Fran's signature was strong and unflinching.

Debbie Burns, the day nurse, appeared at Taylor's bedside holding the white eyelet gown that Fran had brought from home earlier in the day. She maneuvered the fabric deftly around the tubes and monitor wires, knowing they would soon be removed. She opened the drawer where the baby's belongings were kept and, from the multicolored jumble of tiny accessories, she chose a pale yellow pair of socks and a matching hair ribbon. She didn't ask anyone else's opinion. They had more important things on their minds.

With the baby dressed and the necessary papers signed, Fran and Carey found themselves in the conference room once again. Sharon had asked them to leave the nursery, and Gene agreed. Both believed there are certain things no parent should have to watch. Sharon took a few steps toward the warmer, then turned suddenly and walked out of the room, as if remembering a pressing appointment. Her change of direction was not cold feet, it only looked that way. As she approached the warmer, she remembered Randy's voice as it had sounded earlier in the afternoon when he handed her the committee's decision and asked, "Are you going to be okay?" If she looked that bad, she decided, she had best do something about it and turned toward the rest room to apply some lipstick and blusher. There is no point in making other people feel bad, she thought, because you look like you're suffering.

When her face was safely in place, she walked back to Taylor and, with Debbie's help, she began the process of making the baby as presentable as she had just made herself. Wincing slightly, as if feeling the pinch against their own skin, they pulled the tape that held the heart and breathing monitor wires in place. Then they slid the intravenous needles out of her skin, rubbing the lingering puncture spots lightly with their fingers. When there was nothing left to remove but the breathing tube Debbie began shaking slightly. "I've never taken a baby off a ventilator while she's looking at me," she said in a voice as uncertain as her hands. "I can't do it."

"Debbie, just give her the morphine," Sharon said. "I'll take her off the ventilator."

The morphine injection didn't take full effect for fifteen minutes. When Sharon was certain that the baby would not feel the pain of suffocation, she slid the plastic tube from her mouth. Taylor began sucking softly on her hand, the first time she could do that since the moment she was born.

Debbie wrapped the infant in the blankets that had been brought from the home she would never see. At 6:20 in the evening, as families around the city were sitting down to dinner, Debbie lifted Taylor from her warmer, walked with her across the hall to the conference room, and placed her in Fran's arms. Fran and Carey had asked their families to wait in the hallway, and when Debbie left the room, they were alone with their daughter for the first time.

Fran cradled her, then Carey, then Fran. They touched her hands and her feet where the tubes had been, places they couldn't touch before. They told her they loved her and that her brother, Jake, was waiting to see her. Fran nestled her chin on Taylor's head, an unconscious echo of the picture of mother and daughter that looked down from the wall across from the couch.

Fifteen minutes passed before Carey kissed first Taylor then Fran on the top of their heads, then opened the door and motioned to their waiting parents. By that point, the baby was gasping for air. It wasn't the horrible sound they had feared, just very sad. Her breaths were like short, sudden punctuation marks, spaced further and further apart. Then the breaths stopped. Carey's father went across the hall and returned with Sharon, who placed her fingers along the side of Taylor's neck, looking for a pulse. There was none. Sharon took the baby from Fran and walked out of the room. At the door she turned and looked back at the family. "I'm very, very sorry," she said.

Armando

While Fran and Carey were saying their last good-byes to Taylor, Armando Dimas was upstairs in the Neuro Intermediate Unit, learning how to swallow. In the two weeks since he had arrived at Hermann, he had become a tiny bit less helpless. Although he still could not breathe, move, or feel anything below his neck, he had learned to mouth words once his breathing tube was removed from his mouth and placed in an opening in his throat. His speech was completely without sound, and it took the most patient of observers to read his lips correctly. But this was a small triumph over his paralysis, and he used his new power to indicate that mere speech was not enough. Among his first sentences were "When can I eat?" and "How about water?"

Given the extent of his injuries, it was unclear if he would ever be able to do either. That was what Dahlia Harper, a speech therapist, had come to his room to find out. She had been to visit once before, when Armando began demanding to eat and drink through more than just a tube in his arm. During that first session Dahlia had fed him tiny ice chips to test his swallow reflex and make sure that liquid did not run into his lungs. He could feel each chip in his mouth, cold and brittle, a sensation remembered from the days when ice was hardly this extraordinary. He cradled the chip in his tongue until it melted, then waited as it dripped toward the entrance to his throat, cold and clean. He expected the familiar feeling of icy liquid sliding down and into his empty stomach, but that feeling never came. Between his mouth and his belly the coldness stopped. If he concentrated, he could still feel the dripping, or he thought he could, but he couldn't feel the cold. One other thing to get used to.

He didn't bother explaining any of this to Dahlia. He simply opened when she said to open and closed when she said to close and did his best to swallow when she asked him to swallow. "Good gag reflex," Dahlia wrote after that first visit. "Good lingual and labial movement. Weak but adequate chew. No visible signs of problems with onset of swallow. *However*—only small individual ice chips used."

"Next time, we'll try real food," she told him as she left the room.

True to her word, Dahlia arrived for this visit looking like a room service waiter at a bizarre health spa, bearing a tray filled with samples of nearly a dozen foods and drinks of varying viscosity: apple juice, milk, water, ice cream, chocolate pudding, Jell-O.

"Let's take these one at a time," she told him, positioning the tray out of his direct line of vision so he would be a little less disappointed if she were forced by his limitations to stop the test. It must be awful, she thought, to stare expectantly at a cup of ice cream only to watch it taken away.

She began with the juice, pouring a small amount on a spoon and tilting it into his mouth. He swallowed, smacked his lips, and smiled. Dahlia asked him to open as wide as he could and saw that his mouth was empty. A few more spoonfuls, and she was satisfied. It was time for the Jell-O. Armando was never a fan of Jell-O, but he didn't complain as Dahlia put a tiny dab to his lips. This was more difficult than the apple juice because he had to use his tongue to help move the morsel from the spoon. He did so without too much trouble, then pressed the cherry-flavored dot against his front teeth with his tongue to make it melt. He gulped again and opened his mouth without prompting. It was empty. He was able to swallow.

As the test proceeded through the ice cream and chocolate pudding, Dahlia warned Armando that this small success did not mean he would be allowed immediately the tamales and burritos that his family had been bringing to his bedside since he first entered the hospital. Hearing that news, his mood, which had been better than at any time since he arrived at Hermann, suddenly changed. His smiles at each sweet spoonful were the first his nurses had seen. But suddenly his familiar scowl was back again. Dahlia understood. She knew how powerful a sensation taste could be, and she knew, too, that food brought by the family could come to represent warmth and love. She also knew that Armando could choke and die if he tried to swallow solids without first being taught how. "I'm sorry," she said. "Those are the rules for now."

Mrs. Dimas had been standing in a corner of the room watching the test, and Dahlia addressed her for the first time. "He can't eat," she said. "You have to promise you won't give him anything to eat and drink."

Mrs. Dimas's nod did not convince Dahlia, who scribbled yet another note in Armando's chart: "*Do not feed* until speech pathology has evaluated swallowing." It looked like the sort of sign one would hang on the cage of a gastronomically sensitive resident of the local zoo.

It wasn't surprising that Dahlia's order made Armando

cranky. Most things made him cranky in recent days. Physically, he was stronger than anyone had anticipated when he first arrived. Every so often the staff asked him what he wanted them to do if his heart stopped beating, but each time they asked, it was more apparent that his heart had no intention of doing any such thing. He had had only one episode of heart problems since he entered the hospital, and that had resolved itself before anyone could do anything about it. He continued to run fevers as high as 104 degrees, but David MacDougall believed that was not because he was sick but because his body's thermostat was out of whack. He also had persistent lung infections, though they were not nearly as severe as those that were plaguing Patrick. In short, he didn't have any problem that seemed likely to kill him.

The challenge to his caretakers was to maintain that status quo. As the bullet entered his neck, it short-circuited nearly every automatic body function. His loss of muscle tone, for instance, meant there was less support for his veins and arteries, making it harder for them to bring blood and oxygen to his organs and limbs. Similarly, his inability to breathe meant he couldn't do such simple things as clear his throat or cough, allowing secretions to accumulate in his lungs and making him susceptible to pneumonia.

The daily tasks of changing his position to improve his circulation and suctioning his lungs to remove secretions were made more complicated by Armando's poor grasp of English and the fact that he consistently fought his caretakers. What he lacked in physical strength he made up for with his ability to drive everyone around him crazy. To get the attention of the staff, he learned to make a high-pitched chirping sound with his mouth that could be heard up and down the hall. He used this personal paging system almost constantly—moments after a nurse had left the room he would start calling for help again—and someone always responded, just in case this call was really an emergency. It never was. "Move my head up" and "My body should be straighter" were typical requests. He asked to have his mouth suctioned as often as every three minutes when the usual schedule called for suctioning about once an hour. The nurses tried to rig a spittoon for him by taping a cup to the railing of his bed, within range of his mouth. He hated that system and replaced it with one of his own, which consisted of spitting directly at his least favorite nurses whenever they came within range. This made him a less than popular patient.

The staff understood, from textbooks and experience, why Armando acted the way he did. The bullet in his spine had robbed him of control over even the tiniest choices of his life. If his cheek itched, he could not scratch it, if the mood struck, he could not lean on his left side rather than his right. He couldn't cross his legs, wiggle his toes, not to mention change the channel on the television set or turn off the overhead light. In his old life he would have ogled and whistled at the attractive women who marched in and out of his room all day. Now, as they dressed and undressed him and handled his body like it was another piece of hospital equipment, he fantasized about being able to feel the water on his skin as they washed his limbs, and of being able to reach up to bat their hands away so he could finish the task himself.

But he couldn't do that, or anything else for that matter, and he took out his frustration and fear by making their lives at least a modicum as miserable as his own. The staff expected this, but that didn't make him any easier to handle. When Hazel Mitchell stepped onto the unit to do her periodic review of the charges on

Armando's chart, she was met by a chorus of nurses asking only half in jest, "Did you come to take him away?"

In theory, doctors and nurses are not supposed to dislike their patients, but that is just a theory. Some patients are simply difficult to like. "Some are easier to get along with than others," David MacDougall confessed one afternoon while discussing the Armando problem. "As a physician you're not supposed to favor one over the other. Realistically I'm not sure you can honestly say that you don't. You hope it evens out, the person you like more maybe some other doctor might not pay as much attention to and will give more attention to someone you don't like as much."

Armando did in fact have a few champions, and one of them was David MacDougall, who admired his patient's surprising determination to survive. Another was Mary Coffey, Armando's occupational therapist, who was amused and intrigued by the very thing that so angered his nurses—his resolute crankiness. Some of her affection took root in the fact that she was one of the few people at Hermann who could put him in a better mood. She is the unceasingly chipper type, and her exercise sessions were the only part of his endless, monotonous day that Armando truly enjoyed. It didn't take him long to memorize the simple routine, designed to move every muscle in his body. They started with the parts he could move himself. She would place her hand against his cheek, and he would turn his head toward the pressure, exercising his neck with the resistance. Occasionally Mary also applied mild jolts of electricity to his neck, causing contractions that might also strengthen the muscles. This type of exercise was not usual for a quadriplegic, but Mary's instructions from the neurosurgeons remained the same as they were during the first session in the ICU—she could use whatever approach she thought might help because nothing she did could hurt.

They moved from neck turns to shoulder shrugs: "Up and down, up and down." And she would keep her hands on his upper arms and help each shrug along, making him feel as though he really could move. Then came the chest exercises: "Cave it in, pull it out, cave it in, pull it out," with Mary's hands doing most of the work. After that he didn't even pretend to be able to help, but simply watched as she worked her way down his body. The arms, the wrists, the fingers. Move each joint up and down, side to side, circle to the left, then back to the right. The hips, the knees, the ankles, the toes. Ten to fifteen repetitions each. Sometimes he fell asleep but most of the time he looked on, fascinated, at the sight of his body moving without him feeling a thing. It was as if it belonged to someone else. For each forty-five-minute session, that someone else was Mary.

Over the weeks she helped him to do things the textbooks said he couldn't do, such as sitting in a chair. For nearly a month after he was shot, he lay basically flat in his bed, which the human body is not designed to do. In that position, gravity stretches the body out until the lungs become full of stale secretions, and the joints become stiff beyond repair. But for someone like Armando, the dangers of lying down have to be weighed against those of sitting up. His weak muscle tone made it likely that his blood pressure would plummet if his head were raised too far above the level of his heart, causing him to pass out. As Mary explained it, "All the blood just rushes out of their head right down to their feet."

One morning, however, she arrived at his room to find a note in the chart from David saying it was time to try to get Armando out of bed. She found the doctor in the hallway later that afternoon and asked if he really meant what he had written. "How are we going to keep up his diaphragm?" she asked. "How are we going to hold up his head?"

David's answer was much the same as it had been when Mary first asked, weeks earlier, what she was supposed to do with Armando. "He's come through so far," he said. "I think we should give this a try."

One morning in late August Mary did exactly that. She asked Dawn Semner, a friend and a physical therapist, to come help because she was concerned about trying alone. They rolled a padded blue wheelchair into his room, placed it by his bed, and explained what they were going to do. "This chair lies flat, like a bed," Mary told him, "and that's how we're going to start. Then we'll raise you up a little at a time to see what your body can tolerate."

She and Dawn spent nearly twenty minutes wrapping Armando's limbs with ace bandages to help keep his blood pressure up. They slipped thick support hose over his calves, wound more ace bandages around his thighs, and cinched an abdominal binder around his middle. When he was fully mummified, they enlisted the aid of two other nurses, and each of the women took hold of a corner of the sheet on which Armando lay. At the count of three they heaved the sheet like a stretcher and deposited Armando onto the reclining wheelchair.

Mary took a few moments to catch her breath. Armando's blood pressure monitor showed a respectable 112 over 68. Biting her lower lip, Mary raised the back of the chair to an angle of 40 degrees, about the height of two pillows, and the blood pressure readings barely changed. More confident, Mary raised the chair back further, to an angle of 60 degrees, and lowered the foot rest by about the same amount, so that Armando looked like he was sitting in a slightly reclining dentist's chair. His blood pressure was 108 over 70, still acceptable. He said it felt warm but was not lightheaded or dizzy, and his vision wasn't blurred, which would have been signs that his brain wasn't getting enough blood. Armando's first trip to the chair lasted about an hour, and his blood pressure stayed stable throughout. It was not a perfect session, mostly because the standard-size wheelchair was far too big for him. Because there was no headguard, his head flopped toward one side while his body listed toward the other. Mary and Dawn temporarily wedged him in with towels so that he didn't tilt quite as dramatically. At one point they even tied his head to the back board of the chair with a piece of gauze, but he looked so miserable that they quickly removed it.

Equipment problems aside, Mary was pleased with the session. Once her patient was safely back in his bed, she summarized the morning's activities in his chart. "Excellent sitting attempt," she wrote. "Abdominal binder does not provide significant diaphragmatic support to assist this ventilator dependent Pt. Pt. has poor head control. Will work on head control and neck strengthening activities."

It took her several weeks to realize that her atypical affection for Armando sprang largely from the fact that he was teaching her so much. She had only been at Hermann for two years when she met him, and her work experience before that consisted of one year at a private rehabilitation clinic in her native Cape Cod. She chose her profession because a vocational test in high school said she would be happiest as a forest ranger, a commercial artist, or an occupational therapist. She likes to draw, but not enough to do it all day, and she likes trees, but not enough to work with them full-time. She didn't know what an occupational therapist was and asked her mother and two sisters, both of whom are nurses, and her father, who is a doctor. The description appealed to her, and she began training after high school.

Working with Armando made her certain she had made the right choice. It also taught her how far she had come from the nervous student she had been when she first started to work with patients. Over those years she had reached the point where fates such as Armando's didn't tear her apart, didn't keep her up at night thinking, "That could have been me." In the early days, the thought of the life Armando faced made Mary want to flee. But she has learned to distance herself emotionally from the ruined lives she sees every day. She had no urge to flee from Armando, and her ability to deal coolly with this devastated patient made her feel relieved.

"You see this tragic thing and you think, 'This should keep me awake at night,' " she once explained. "It used to keep me awake, so I must have really changed. I've learned to separate myself so I can sleep at night.

"You have to keep emotional distance," she said. "That's hard but it's also necessary so that I don't lose my objectivity or effectiveness. You have to take the attitude, 'I'm glad it's not me. I'm sorry it's you. But let's get to work.' My role is to teach independence and avoid dependence, on me or anyone else."

Working with Armando not only taught Mary about herself, but also provided an education about the institution where she worked. Before taking this job, she had looked at other hospitals and rehabilitation centers. Most of them were in better financial shape than this one, and, oddly, that was part of the reason she chose

Hermann. "In college we were trained as occupational therapists," she explains. "We knew exactly what needed to be done. But then you get to the reality of the hospital, and you realize you can't do everything you've been taught to do. You don't have four or five hours a day for each patient, and you don't have an unlimited budget, so you have to explore every available avenue. You have to be resourceful. There are a lot of things they don't tell you about in school."

While some people might have been depressed by that shock of reality, Mary found herself challenged. "I'm here to see what I can do with the least amount of equipment," she says. In the case of Armando, she gradually developed a host of ambitious plans, all of them designed to give him something to do with his days and, eventually, with his life. She wanted to teach him to use a "mouth stick"—a long slender stick with a mouthpiece at one end that can be used to do tasks usually done by fingers, tasks such as pressing computer keyboards and remote control panels or writing on a chalkboard. Time and patience could eventually translate those abilities into a job. At the least he could learn to play games, like blowing Velcro-covered darts, so he would have something to do besides watch television and drive his nurses up the wall.

All these plans depend on the proper equipment, however, and that equipment has to be paid for. Mary knew how unlikely it was that Hermann could simply give a charity patient these life-enhancing extras. Over the years she had learned to choose her battles carefully, and as the weeks passed and Armando showed ever-increasing potential, she decided that this was one of those battles. She knew she would have to start slowly, one step at a time. Her first skirmish would be over the simplest, most basic part of the problem. Without proper head control, Armando would never be able to learn to do much of anything, and he would never achieve the head control if he was all but swallowed by his wheelchair. It was time to fight the bureaucracy for a new chair.

The Cost of Care

Every Thursday at 9:30 in the morning a group of Hermann middle managers and staff gather in a cramped windowless office to discuss all those patients who are unable to pay their bills. Hazel Mitchell always tries to attend, as does Lee Zacharias, the director of Social Work, and as many of her staff members as are free and have a relevant patient on their caseload that week.

The meetings are run by Willene Guttenberger, the director of Patient Financial Services, an imposing, authoritative woman who on this particular morning wasted no time getting down to business. On the table in front of her was a computer printout of the forty uninsured and underinsured patients at Hermann who had together run up bills of $2,356,232 over the previous week. Eight of those patients had exhausted their Medicaid, at a loss of $441,105 to the hospital. One had only limited private insurance and an unpaid bill of $31,521. Twenty-four were in financial class U, meaning their application for insurance was pending, and together those patients owed $1,654,848. Seven were in financial class R, which means they had no insurance at all. Together they owed $228,758. That didn't even include the fourteen uninsured patients who had been admitted by helicopter during the summer and in the past week alone had run up a total bill of $1,125,090. One of those was Armando Dimas.

"Okay, let's start," Willene said, flipping through the green-and-white striped computer sheets.

First on the list was Mr. Rodriguez, a quadriplegic like Armando, also uninsured, also from Mexico, also in need of years of rehabilitation with little expectation that any of it would work.

"He's keeping us busy," said Valerie Buffam, the pale, overworked social worker who was sharing the case with Cindy Walker. "We decided we would keep him here and rehabilitate him, so we sent him over to the rehab unit, and he told them he wanted to go back to Mexico. So we said, 'Fine, we'll help you do that, too.' So we called the consulate, and they sent someone over, and he told that consulate man he wanted to stay here. So we started all over again."

As Valerie Buffam spoke, Cindy entered the room, mumbled her apologies, and launched right in with her opinion. "You can't let him vacillate. He can't say he wants to stay here, he wants to go back to Mexico, he wants to stay here. We may have to be more definite. Tell him he's leaving, period, and that his mother will have to go to the consulate and get the papers. Say, 'We will give you the wheelchair, we will get you on the plane.' If he refuses to leave, we'll send him to the consulate, which will refuse to take him, and then we'll bring him back here, but at least we gave it a try."

Valerie Buffam shook her head slightly and extended an outstretched palm toward Cindy as if to cede that responsibility to her. Before she could speak, Willene interrupted, fine-tuning Cindy's plan.

"We have to have one of our translators there when you tell him," Willene said. "Call the consulate, but have one of our own translators, too. We can't depend on the consulate to do our work for us. We don't know what these people really are saying.

"Where does his mother live?"

"Here in Houston."

Willene made a note on her computer printout. "If they are eligible for care at Harris County, they are not eligible for charity care here," she said, without looking up, in a voice that made it clear it was time to discuss the next case.

"That would be Mrs. Connor, the one waiting for a heart transplant," Valerie Buffam said. "Nothing's changed. The team still says she won't survive without one."

"We're going to have this lady here until she dies or until the family raises the seventy-five thousand dollars and can transfer her to St. Luke's for a transplant."

"We can tell the family to contact their congressman," Cindy offered. "In an election year it's amazing what a congressman can do."

"We can't tell them that officially," Willene said, "but it's worth a try. Next."

The list was depressing and long.

The nineteen-year-old college student who fell off a balcony backward and broke his neck. He could be transferred to a hospital near his parents in Dallas, but someone, namely Hermann Hospital, would have to pay to get him there. Five minutes were spent discussing whether he should make that trip by ambulance or airplane. The decision was that at a cost of $650, the six-hour ambulance ride was cheaper than the one-hour airplane trip, mostly because his stretcher would not fit on the airplane unless four first-class seats were removed.

"Next," Willene said.

The unemployed heroin addict, who tested positive for the virus that causes AIDS, who had no insurance, and needed sixty-three days of amphotericin, the same tricky medication that rules Patrick's life. The drug can only be given intravenously, and the man's doctors were afraid that on the days between treatments he would use the semipermanent tube in his arm as a convenient way to mainline. The question: Since he was dying of AIDS anyway and the AIDS was a result of his drug addiction, did he have to be given an expensive treatment for a secondary infection? The decision: Yes. Hermann could not make moral judgments about who deserved treatment. Did he have to be kept in the hospital during the treatment to protect him from himself? No, Hermann's responsibility did not extend that far. Next.

The thirty-three-year-old woman with Krohn's disease, a debilitating malfunction of the digestive system. She has two children, and her husband owns a small trucking company. One of the cutbacks he was forced to make recently was his health insurance. The family makes too much money to qualify for the Harris County hospital, but not enough to pay what promise to be sky-high bills. "Now, *these* are the kind of people we're here for," said Willene, her mind still on the heroin addict discussed a few minutes before. "People who otherwise will fall through the cracks. We can count them under charity care." Next.

The one-year-old boy who was using his bed as a trampoline and missed the edge of the mattress, cracking his skull. His mother, a housekeeper at Methodist Hospital, had dropped her dependent coverage three weeks before the accident, and her own employer would not admit her son because he was not insured.

"I think she has sixty days to reinstate her insurance," Lee suggested.

"We can even pay the premium," Willene said. "I've paid people's insurance before." Next.

At the end of the list, a place determined by chance, not significance, was Armando Dimas. Cindy reviewed his tale for those few who didn't already know it. "It's been a month," she said. "He still doesn't want to be made DNR."

"What happens if he starts asking us to turn off his ventilator?" Valerie Buffam said.

"I don't think he's concerned with getting off the ventilator. I think what he wants most of all is to eat," Cindy answered.

"What has he cost us so far?" Willene asked, bringing the meeting back on track.

Cindy handed her Hazel's latest tally, and Willene took a few seconds to scan the page. "Nearly $60,000 in three weeks, not that bad," she said, but she did not look at all happy.

"We tried to send him back to Madisonville," Cindy offered. "No success yet."

"The most gracious thing that could happen to him is to die here," Willene said.

"He's not going to die though," said Cindy. "He's not going to die. You should see him. He looks great."

"Keep me up to date," Willene said, and the meeting was over.

SEPTEMBER

Patrick

To no one's surprise and everyone's frustration, Patrick was admitted to Hermann early one autumn morning when he should have been starting school. His central line had finally blocked completely. At bedtime the night before, Oria had hooked her son to the omnipresent bag of liquid nutrition. Come sunrise, the bag was still full, its contents stalled like beach traffic on the freeway, unable to penetrate the clogged lifeline.

At first Patrick thought this visit would be a short and easy one. The plan was to drip a clot dissolver through the line for three hours, as they had done during the summer, and then try the nutrients again. But, as usual, nothing about Patrick's treatment was easy. Despite repeated tries, the bag of TPN remained full, and Patrick spent the night on the pediatrics floor.

The next morning, a chest X ray showed that the central line, still securely stitched into his heart, was all but fully obstructed. The news, upsetting as it was to Patrick, was devastating to Javier. He sat slumped in the office of his department chairman, Jan Van Eys, holding, but not drinking, a cup of coffee and asking the older, wiser man what he should do.

"Should we try another surgery?" he asked, not meeting his mentor's eye.

"We've talked about this before."

"I know all the arguments against inserting a new line, but I don't think we have any other option."

"If you keep asking the question, that can only mean you are hoping for a different answer."

Javier had no response.

Dr. Van Eys worries about Javier. The older doctor earned much of his flop of white hair worrying about his own patients, but along the way he learned that there are two types of doctorly concern. The first kind, the bad kind, is when concern is really a means of control. Many doctors who choose to deal with severely ill patients, he believes, come to need the ego stroke of helping a patient when all others have given up. Their patients become a scorecard, and each setback or death becomes a sign of the doctor's failure. The second kind of concern is closer to true compassion. These doctors feel the need to take the pain of their patients upon themselves, telling them, in effect, "Don't worry, I'll do the worrying for you."

There is a suture-fine line between empathy and self-destruction, and Jan Van Eys often worries that Javier has crossed it. "I like Javier immensely, he's a wonderful doctor, and he'll learn," Van Eys says. "I hope he learns before he burns out."

Roseanne Aceves worries about her husband, too. Since he opened CHOSEN, Javier has become even quieter at home, exhausted from the emotion of particularly bad days. His monologues to Rosie used to be his way of sorting out his thoughts, but over the years he has stopped talking about work when he is home. Instead, he disappears into the workshop in the garage where he hammers and saws and builds things he doesn't need, in the hope that working with his hands will make his brain shut up.

Sometimes his workshop is too distracting. One February evening, when Patrick was in the hospital yet again, Javier came home, exhausted, and decided to fix the shingles on the side of his house. "I have to do something with my hands," he told Rosie as he went to fetch a hammer and a saw to use in the dark. Less than an hour later, he walked back in, holding his bloodied left arm above his shoulder and applying pressure with his other hand. He had cut off the tip of his middle finger, an accident that he admits a Freudian analyst could endlessly dissect. Within an hour he was on an operating table at Hermann having his finger, which he had salvaged and packed in ice, sewn back on.

Rosie saw the accident as a physical sign of the emotional torture her husband was inflicting on himself. "What happened to you?" she asked him. "You used to go to work and be happy and look forward to the next day. What's come over you? Why are you hurting yourself this way? Do you really need to be a masochist? Do you really want to do this?"

Her prodding was gentle and helpful, leading Javier to face questions he had been avoiding since CHOSEN began. "I just feel there's a need, and I'm the one to fill it," he told her. "But I'm less sure than I used to be that I can do this for the rest of my life."

That was a rare admission of pain. Javier rarely takes time out to worry about himself. There was no room in his day for that—not with all the worrying he was doing about Patrick and the question that wouldn't go away.

The person he went to most often with that question was Dr. Richard Andrassy, the chief of pediatric surgery at Hermann, who had inserted many of Patrick's central lines and who would insert the next one if there were to be a next one. Their conversations rarely went well.

While Javier's relationship with Jan Van Eys is warm and avuncular, he feels only distance from Dr.

Andrassy. The surgeon came to Hermann in 1985, taking over for Dr. Stan Dudrick, the man who practically created the science of feeding patients like Patrick. Doctors Andrassy and Dudrick are close friends, and Dr. Dudrick's picture hangs on Dr. Andrassy's wall. Javier finds himself glancing away from the framed photograph every time he enters the room, as if ashamed that he is somehow failing to use properly the tools of Dr. Dudrick.

But the picture is only the smallest of many reasons why Javier dislikes visits to Dr. Andrassy's office. It irks Javier that he has to go to that office in the first place because the more senior surgeon won't come to him. At nearly all the meetings about Patrick, Dr. Andrassy is noticeably absent. Sometimes he'll send a nurse or assistant in his place, but only sometimes, and he almost never attends himself. He will speak one-on-one with Javier whenever the pediatrician calls, and he is always cordial and interested, but he rarely initiates the discussion himself.

What Dr. Andrassy has never explained to Javier is his philosophy about meetings—specifically, that nearly all of them are a waste of time. If he had explained it, his reasoning would have sounded something like this:

"I think sometimes some things don't get done because of meetings. You have meetings instead of doing anything. And the answer to this meeting is to have another meeting and then have a subcommittee instead of just saying, 'This is what we're going to do.'

"I purposely don't show up a lot. I think it's a waste of time because I know in the long run what it's going to boil down to. We can sit there and talk for three hours and in the end someone will ask me, 'Can you do it?' and my answer will be, 'Yes, if you want me to do it I'll do it.' For that, you don't need a meeting.

"Take Patrick. Every month we decide we aren't going to do anything, and then I'll get a call saying, 'Let's have a conference.' Well, the conference mentality is you have twenty people sitting around a table, and nobody wants to say, 'Let's let him die.' Everybody says, 'Yes, we know he's going to die,' but nobody will say, 'Let's let him die.' So at some point I say, and I make sure everybody hears my words, I say, 'Patrick is going to die. He may die from the operation. If he doesn't die from the operation, he's going to die sometime in the future.' I make it perfectly clear, time and time again, that we are talking about a major operation. But when he really starts to deteriorate, they always come to me and say, 'Will you give it a try?' Of course I'll give it a try, that's what I do. Maybe I should say, 'No, this is pointless.' I know some surgeons would say that, but I believe that if the family and the doctor ask me to operate, then I operate, and I do the best job I can. They know that, so they put it back in my lap. It's much easier to do something than nothing, particularly if something means passing it to someone else.

"No one understands, that's why I don't show up. They think I'm just being a pain in the butt."

All the conversations that Javier had with Dr. Andrassy were almost identical. Javier would ask if a new line should be put in, the surgeon would recite the risks of opening Patrick's chest another time, and Javier would write a note in Patrick's chart summarizing the conversation. ("Discussed surgery option with Dr. Andrassy. Because of multiple previous surgeries replacement of line would be technically very difficult and hazardous. Do not think patient would survive such a hazardous procedure. Would not recommend further surgery.") Then, days later, he would raise the subject again.

Jan Van Eys was right. Javier wanted a different answer. Rising from his chair and tossing his coffee cup in the trash, he set out down the hall in search of one.

Finding Dr. Andrassy, Javier again raised the idea of replacing the current line with a clean one. The surgeon, as usual, was not optimistic. "The risk of the operation itself is extremely high," he said. "Even if he survives, there's no guarantee the new line will ever work. It will clot off rapidly, and what would we have accomplished?"

"I know all this," Javier said. "But what's the alternative?"

They both knew the answer, of course. Patrick would have to be fed through peripheral IV tubes, the type that are inserted into the visible, accessible veins of the arms and legs. It was an inefficient method, which is why the boy had been given a central line in the first place. Each peripheral IV would clot and become useless within hours or days, and another site would have to be found. Patrick's veins were already as fragile as onion skin after years of overuse. It wouldn't take long, Javier knew, before there were no more places to pierce with an IV needle, and his patient would starve to death.

Surgical replacement of the line was hardly a guarantee, but it was something in place of nothing, action in place of inaction, a sliver of hope in place of helpless resignation. Over the years, Javier had held countless discussions, in conference rooms and over coffee, about the tendency of doctors to fight too hard and to do too much. He always spoke in favor of realizing the limits of medicine and being able to let go. Had it been as easy as that, however, all those conferences and conversations would not have been necessary and the rationality of care would not be a question so complex that Lin could spend four years studying it.

Faced, finally, with the choice he had been inching toward for years, Javier could not simply let Patrick die. Yet he couldn't insist that Dr. Andrassy operate, either. He left the surgeon's office and spent a distracted afternoon seeing a parade of patients in the clinic. By dinnertime, he decided to do what no one had done for fifteen years. He decided to ask Patrick.

Armando

If being able to eat was truly Armando's fondest wish, as he insisted it was, then he was a very happy young man by Labor Day. It took most of August before Dahlia's daily tests ruled out any physical reason why he couldn't eat and several more weeks for her to teach him how to best use his functioning mouth muscles to help the chewing and swallowing process. He began by sipping clear liquids through a straw. Soon he was eating everything in sight. His mother, who had sat helplessly by his bed from 9 A.M. to 7 P.M. every day, saw his ability to eat as a chance to reenter his life, and each morning she came laden with plates of homemade tamales and burritos that she had cooked the night before. She fed these offerings to him with her hands, ripping off each bite and placing it gently in his mouth, then patting his lips with a napkin after each swallow.

He could talk, too. At the end of August, the breathing tube in his throat was enhanced with a device called a talking trach. With proper training, patients fitted with this device can collect air in their lungs, then force it slowly through the double rings of the tube to produce a breathless, hoarse sound. Armando was a surprisingly quick learner, and it wasn't more than a week before he was bossing the nurses around in a throaty whisper. Most of his orders and complaints were suddenly given in English. The staff wasn't sure whether two months in the hospital listening mostly to his second language had improved his skills or whether he was always more fluent in English than he had let on, preferring to eavesdrop on his caretakers.

He was even making progress physically. When Mary touched his right shoulder, he could usually feel the pressure, and every once in a while he also felt pressure when, as a test, she pressed her fingernail into the soles of his feet. He complained periodically of "pain" in his lower back and when Mary alternately held a cold towel and then a hot one to his skin he could tell which was which three-fifths of the time. Getting him into his wheelchair was no longer the production it had been weeks earlier. He could be placed directly into something akin to full sitting position and stay there without any discomfort for more than two hours.

That was the good news. The bad news was that his wheelchair was still too big, his head control was nonexistent, and Mary had little hope that any of his physical and emotional progress could be translated into vocational ability until those problems were fixed. She tried stuffing pillows against his sides, like packing in an oversized crate, to keep his body straight. When that didn't work, she added blankets and seat cushions from the visitors area, anything she could find. She rolled towels and wedged them behind his neck to keep his head from flopping from side to side. Finally she found three foam belts, used to strap patients down when they are wheeled around on gurneys, and she used one each at his head, his shoulders, and his legs. It was a technique she had occasionally used to align comatose patients, but this patient could look her in the eye as she bound him to his chair and doing so became the worst part of her day.

"We might as well gag him, too," she said. "It's got to be a scary feeling, and it doesn't do any good for his orthopedic alignment, either."

She had certainly tried to find him a better chair. The pediatric versions were too small. The specially designed versions used by the neurology department were equally unacceptable, because when the headrests on those were raised, the footrests automatically lowered, and there were days when Armando could not tolerate having his feet down on the ground. She tried to borrow a chair from the rehabilitation center down the block, perhaps one that they were preparing to throw out, but they didn't have enough for their own patients. She talked to Cindy and to Hazel, who were sympathetic but not encouraging. "We can't just buy him a custom-made wheelchair," Cindy told her. "We have to face the fact that we can't afford him as it is."

Over the weeks, the saga of Armando's chair made Mary steadily angrier. She knew all about Hermann's finite resources, but she believed Armando's needs deserved a larger portion of those resources than he was being given. "You have this totally, totally debilitated man whose only chance to interact with the world is to get him equipment that he could have control over," she responded to Cindy. "It's so annoying that this man was admitted with open arms when he was a donor, and now that we have to treat him as a man, we're hemming and hawing."

One day she carefully put this frustration on two pages of single-spaced paper, which she then mailed to Hazel Mitchell.

"I am writing to you in regards to funding sources available to purchase a wheelchair and head support for Armando Dimas," she wrote. "Mr. Dimas is a quadriplegic patient with no resources and extensive equipment needs. We have reviewed his essential needs and have come up with the following recommendations and rationales:

"Rehab Goals—achieving limited head control in gravity eliminated plane, prevention of neck deformity, prevention of glenohumeral subluxation, prevention of skin compromise, and preservation of passive range of motion in the upper and lower extremities to prevent further deformity.

"Mr. Dimas has progressed quickly through a progressive sitting program, achieving a 90° angle without distress. He utilizes foam seat cushions, abdominal binder, and ted hose. Presently, he has been utilizing a variety of highback wheel chairs and 'Neuro' chairs to sit for 3–4 hours daily. In these chairs he requires pillows, foam, and towel rolls to prop up feet, support elbows and hands, and to provide head alignment. The head support has been a primitive system of lateral and occipital towel rolls, and a forehead strap resulting in alignment consistently less than optimal. This appropriate alignment and support is an absolute necessity before sufficient strengthening and compensation can be achieved with eventual progression toward mouthstick activities.

"This patient obviously has many expensive equipment requirements to achieve function; however, his financial resources are severely limited, if not nonexistent, and his family support is marginal. With these limitations in mind there remains the necessities required to maintain this man's existence. The ventilator, tracheostomy, gastrostomy feedings are obviously on top of the list; however, from a rehabilitation standpoint, a correct fitting wheelchair and head support is also a necessity to achieve the aforementioned goals in addition to preventing subhuman existence.

"As Hermann Hospital has accepted the responsibility to care for this unfortunate gentleman, we strongly recommend that the hospital consider purchasing or renting a wheelchair and head support in view of the fact that the patient will be a long-term resident of Hermann Hospital and he will be permanently disabled. In addition, the equipment currently available to him is not adequate to prevent deformity."

The letter was accompanied by a list of prices, which Mary had compiled one afternoon when she called every supply company in the telephone book. In her opinion, Armando's minimal needs would include "One Everest and Jennings Reclining Traveler Wheelchair with adjustable arm rests and foot rests. Purchase price $819. Trunk positioners to promote upright posture and prevent musculoskeletal deformity, purchase price $251.20. Spongy-wedge head support, purchase price $235.75. Total price, including a 20 percent discount from Abbey Medical—$1,305.95."

Interoffice mail moves slowly at Hermann, and Hazel did not receive the letter until a week after it was mailed. That happened to be a Thursday morning, the day of the weekly meeting of Willene Guttenberger's nonresource committee. As soon as the committee had gathered, Hazel pulled out the letter, plunked it dramatically on the table, then picked it up gingerly and handed it to her boss, who read it quickly, then passed it on to the person seated to her left. As the pages made their way around the table, Hazel talked nonstop.

"A *letter*," she said. "I never get a *letter*. Usually they just call me and tell me what we need. I didn't know things were so formal around here.

"A letter. Out of the blue. A *two-page* letter. This is ridiculous. It came through the interoffice mail, I just found it in my box."

"In your opinion, does he need a new chair?" Willene Guttenberger asked.

"It's not uncommon for us to use towels or tie patients in," Hazel answered. "As you can see from the letter, the word she uses is 'dehumanized.' Dehumanized. I think that's a little dramatic.

"If the patient really needs something, for the most part I okay it," she said, slowing her words slightly. "There are some people here with the feeling that they've got to go to extremes in their requests. I screen those requests, I prioritize things. They have a tendency to rattle off everything he may possibly need and I say, 'Okay, let's prioritize, what does he *really* need.' And if it's a safety thing or if it's a deformity thing, of course he's going to have it. We will bend over backward whether it's starting him out with it here, hooking him up with the system after he leaves. It's our legal responsibility."

"Does he need that chair?" Willene asked again. "Do we have an old one that can be converted?"

"He could be tied with a towel," Hazel said, but her tone was less angry and hinted at compromise. "People are tied all the time like that. But I see the point. He's alert and awake, and it's different tying up a comatose patient than someone who's alert. So if this will help him from an emotional standpoint, we should do it. This man is not out to lunch, and maybe it *is* dehumanizing, considering most of the ones we tie up are out to lunch, and he's not."

"Understood," Willene said. "Now, how do we keep down the cost?"

Hazel had done some research of her own. "I don't think we need to buy it outright, we can rent it, which Mary doesn't suggest in her letter. I got a quote of seventy-eight dollars a month, including a forty percent discount. Mary had only gotten us a twenty percent discount."

Cindy interrupted. "If he's going to be here for years, do we want to rent forever?"

"That's another thing we should talk about," Hazel said. "I don't think he needs to be here for the rest of his life. I think we need to start talking about transferring him to Bart's."

There were nods of understanding all around the table. This group had had this conversation about other patients before.

Bart is Hermina Bartkowski, and she runs something called the Total Life Care Center on a scruffy sidestreet near downtown Houston. The single-story institutional-looking building, which was originally built as a county school for the handicapped, houses an alternative in health care, a place Hermann sometimes uses to get out from under the financial strain of patients like Armando. Instead of keeping such patients in a high-cost hospital room for the rest of their lives, Hermann pays Bart to care for them. Without Hermann patients, her twenty-two-bed facility for ventilator-dependent patients would probably not stay solvent. Without Bart, Hermann would probably be in even more desperate financial shape.

Bart's is a cheerful place in spite of its grim, utilitarian reason for being. Two finches chirp in a cage by the front door, next to the sunny plant-filled atrium and across from the colorfully furnished recreation area. The hallways are wide and bright. All the rooms are filled with plants, photographs, and stuffed animals—even the rooms of comatose patients who have no idea that the cozy touches are there.

Many who work with Bart call her a saint, a particularly flattering term given the tendency of medical pro-

fessionals toward understatement. As she walks from
room to room in the institution she fought to create, it
is easy to see where the description came from. None of
the twisted bodies or the vacant stares seem to depress
her, or, more accurately, she refuses even to hint at that
depression when there is any chance a patient might
overhear. She speaks to the unresponsive residents as if
they understand every word.

"I thought you were sleeping but you were only fooling," she will singsong in her rich Polish accent to a
baby in a wheelchair, who has had only the barest of
brain function since a severe car accident several
months ago. "You were only fooling me, and I thought
you were asleep.

"You were joking, you were joking," she'll say,
straightening the child's head in his chair. Only after
she's out the door will she whisper, "It can break your
heart."

Bart learned nursing in Poland. She fled that country
in 1973 when she was granted a tourist visa to visit relatives in the United States, and she decided not to go
back. Her husband, a ship's pilot, escaped several years
later, in the coal bin of a freighter. "He almost froze,
but he got out," she says.

In order to work as a nurse in her adopted country,
Bart had to retake the nursing boards some twenty-four
years after she finished nursing school. Her English,
now colorful and affluent, was shaky when she first arrived, and it took her far too long to read each question.
She passed, but barely. For the next ten years she
worked in the intensive care units of several Houston
hospitals, in a nearby rehabilitation center, and as a
home care nurse for ventilator-dependent patients. During those years she slowly formulated her plan.

"When I was working with people at home on a machine, I had the idea," she explains. "The shortage of nurses is so tremendous. It takes five nurses to take care of one patient on three shifts over twenty-four hours, and I thought, 'What a waste.' You could put three patients together in a house and give them a nurse and a nurse's aide, the same number of nurses could take care of three, not one, and the cost could be a third. It's astronomical to take care of one respirator-dependent patient at home, at least twenty-eight thousand, maybe thirty-two thousand dollars per month. I started thinking there had to be a way that makes more sense."

Hospitals and families could not afford to keep these patients, and nursing homes rejected them because they were not insured. What then would make more sense? Her plan was to find a big house, a place that felt like a home, with a backyard and a mix of sun and shade where wheelchairs could be parked depending on the weather. Her facility would not officially be a nursing home because it would not house enough patients, so she would not be constrained by the reams of state rules about nursing homes. The bills would be paid by the hospitals—at rates that seemed like bargains when compared with decades of charges for expensive ICU beds.

"I was the one who had to do this," she says. "I'm not scared of respirators and life support. A lot of nurses are scared of respirators. It's not like the lights are going to blink, and it will stop working, but a tube might fall off and something can go wrong with the machine and that's it. The person can't breathe. The responsibility is very huge. But if you're familiar with the machines, you're not scared.

"Some of these patients need intensive care, but they're stable," she continues. "They can't breathe, but they're stable, and for the stable ones there should be a different kind of life than a cubicle in an ICU or even a bedroom at home where there's nothing but a television and five faces of five nurses on rotating shifts. Some of these people have normal minds. There's nothing wrong with their minds at all. They just can't move."

She had never worked at Hermann and had no contacts there, but on a hunch she wrote a letter that ended up in Willene Guttenberger's hands. Bart happened to pick a moment when Hermann had five lifetime boarders on their neuro floor. Willene inquired what Bart's expected bill would be and learned that each patient transferred to her "dream house" would save the hospital $17,000 per month. After checking her credentials to be certain that this angel wasn't too good to be true, Willene sent two patients to the hastily remodeled single-story house owned by Bart's son. Months later, Hermann offered to send three more patients, and Bart scrambled to buy a second house, lest she spill over the limit that the state defined as a nursing home. The need for two buildings was a sign of her success, but it also defeated her original plan of keeping the patients together in order to cut costs and increase interaction and efficiency. Two houses required two pantries, two kitchens, two supply rooms, two medicine cabinets. It also required that Bart be in two places at once, something even she could not manage to do.

So she adapted her dream a bit, leasing the empty county-owned building that used to be a rehabilitation center. In some ways, the building's former life suited her purposes perfectly. The doubly wide doorways, for instance, could easily accommodate stretchers and wheelchairs. In other ways, the built-ins were absurd, such as the waist-high light switches in every room designed for wheelchair-bound residents with much greater freedom of movement than her patients will ever have. "These people can't flick a light on and off," she said, entering a room and absentmindedly reaching for the switch in its more traditional spot, a mistake she makes countless times each day. "It can be a pain in the neck."

Equally irritating, she says, is the money she had to spend to bring the building up to code. She was now officially a nursing home, something she had vowed never to be, and the fact that she planned to run a homelike facility, with love and field trips and finches by the entrance, did not alter the requirements that the local health department applied to institutions of her size. She didn't mind fixing the roof, which was leaking, or the air-conditioning system, which blew warm air when it blew at all, or replacing the floors where the tiles were cracked or worn. Most of those repairs, along with hours of painting and scrubbing, were done by herself, her twenty-seven-year-old son, and her cousin Christina, a registered nurse from Poland.

What she did mind was work she considered completely irrelevant to her increasingly complicated goal. The rules and regulations, she complained, were created for nursing homes where the patients were mobile. In such places, it makes sense that the water in each room not be hotter than 110 degrees so that the ill and the elderly don't burn themselves accidentally. But her patients could not get to the sink, and they certainly could not turn on the tap. Yet she had to spend $16,000 for a separate water pump that limits the temperature of the faucets in each room.

She also chafed at rules that were designed for facilities much larger than hers. Growing up in a Communist country, she thought she had seen the worst absurdities of bureaucracy until she learned that she could not open the doors until she had established a separate committee for utilization review, infection control, patient care, medical care planning, nursing, education. With only five full-time administrators, each is at least one committee unto his or herself, responsible for holding meetings and filling out appropriate paperwork to document what goes on at those meetings. "We do what we have to do, and don't do what won't be noticed," she jokes. "We do what we have to do to stay open."

That Bart's stays open has become increasingly important to Hermann. Of the two dozen patients in her care at any given time, about one-fourth are being paid for by Hermann, and she saves the hospital up to $70,000 each month. She can do that because she hires people that other facilities will not. In addition to her twenty licensed nurses, she employs between thirty and thirty-five nurse's aides, depending on the number of patients. Many of her workers are recent Polish immigrants, and many of them were doctors or nurses in their homeland who are waiting for certification to allow them to practice in the United States. While they wait for their English to improve enough to pass their boards, they need a paycheck that will allow them to eat. Bart hires them as technicians and nurse's aides, allowing her to provide a quality of care not usually available at such a low cost.

She is proud of the cleanliness of her building and of the thoroughness of her care. Like a cruise director on a luxury ship, she easily recites the services available for all patients, whatever their level of consciousness. "Every day, three meals and a snack, medicines on individual schedule, suctioning whenever needed, physical therapy, of course we have that, we bathe them every day, brush their teeth, dress them. Everybody gets dressed every day, no lying in bed in pajamas, everyone gets out of bed. There is no dignity if you spend every day in bed.

"On Mondays, we weigh the patients, Tuesdays we do nail care, Wednesday, we wash their hair. Thursdays foot care, and on like that. Every day of the week attention is paid to a part of the body. Each nurse has three patients, so she's there constantly. The only time she's not there is when she's bathing somebody else next door, but the minute she finishes that, she has to go back and check the other two. It's a constant vigil. These patients, the ones who can understand, they need to know someone is always there."

At any given time, up to half of Bart's patients can understand. For those who are conscious, there are field trips: the circus, the zoo, shopping at the mall for Christmas gifts. The excursions require weeks of planning. Vans with wheelchair ramps must be ordered, staff schedules must be changed so that there is one attendant to push each wheelchair, the security staff at the day's destination must be informed. Despite the hassle, the trips are the best part of Bart's job. When one early summer trip to the Astrodome was a disappointment because the home team lost, Bart scheduled a late-summer repeat trip and that time the Astros won. Had they lost on the second visit, she would have taken everyone back once more. "I didn't think it was fair that they would lose when my patients were there," she says. "The time they finally won, everybody came back with a huge grin on their face. There's so little I can give them."

She would like to give more, but she resigned herself a long time ago to the fact that she cannot. "I believe we are the givers of care," she says. "Not the givers of life or the givers of health, just the givers of care. The only way to take care of people like that who are heavily, heavily injured is not to feel, 'Why can't I make them better? Maybe if I did this or maybe if I did that.' That used to drive me crazy. But the way to deal with it is to think, 'I am the giver of the best care in the world, and the rest is really not in my hands.' "

In the early years, Willene Guttenberger would have felt guilt pangs at sending the saintly Bart as difficult a burden as Armando. Since then Willene has learned that it is the unruly patients who don't stand a chance against Bart. So far there isn't one she could not calm and tame. Her attitude toward discipline is summed up in her explanation of why she failed only one section of her American nursing boards, the psychology section. The question she remembers best was about a five-year-old boy who slaps his nurse in the face. "The answer they wanted," she says, "was to sit the boy down and ask, 'Why did you do that? Are you scared? Did it make you feel less scared?'

"But that wasn't my answer," she says, folding her hands together and burying them into her lap. "I wrote down that I would hit back." She pauses, waiting for the expected expression of shock. "Don't worry, I wouldn't really hit him. But that was the philosophy of the old country. I wouldn't hit him, but I would let that little five-year-old boy know it isn't okay to slap the nurse. Why should I ask him why he did it? I know why he did it. He's scared and needs to control and vent anger. But that doesn't make it okay to hit. And it doesn't help him get better to let him do things that are bad. I would hug him and calm him too, but first I would make sure he doesn't hit."

With the nursing boards far behind her, that philosophy is the one still followed at Bart's. Just because you're paralyzed, her message goes, doesn't mean you're allowed to be rude. Her first patient was the first test of this approach. He was a lot like Armando, always angry and difficult, and he vented his constant rage at the nursing staff. When the nurses ignored his name-calling, he, too, began to spit at them and became fairly proficient at hitting his targets. So, as part of what Bart calls a "behavior modification program," a towel was placed over his face when he began this unacceptable behavior, an effective measure because he could not move the towel away. It was a harmless piece of cloth—the nurses were careful that it not cover his eyes—and it made its point. It was particularly effective when coupled with a minilecture Bart delivered just after what turned out to be his last spitting session. "We know you lost everything," she said to the veiled figure in the bed. "The one thing you have is your self-respect and you have to keep that. But you don't keep that by acting like an animal. You keep that by acting like a person. The nurses have to clean you and do things for you that your own family wouldn't want to do. They do it because they love you. They care about what happens to you. You don't have to love them back. But don't curse and call them a bitch."

Within a week the young man had apologized to his nurses, and he never spat at them again.

Willene knew all about Bart's stern side. That first patient, after all, had been sent to Bart's by Hermann. A few months in such an environment might do wonders for Armando, she thought. It would certainly do wonders for Hermann. But it would be impossible to transfer him in the foreseeable future, because hospital rules placed a limit on the number of patients Hermann could keep at Bart's at any given time.

The limit of six was an arbitrary number and grew out of the belief that allowing more than that would provide too easy an out and would lessen the motivation to find a way to remove such patients from Hermann's jurisdiction entirely. When Mary wrote her letter to Hazel, the quota of one-half dozen was already met. Either someone would have to change the rules or Armando would have to stay put until one of those six was transferred or died.

"What's his daily cost here?" Willene asked Hazel.

"It's down to about eight hundred ninety dollars a day."

"And what would it be there?"

"About three hundred."

Willene winced.

"We have no other options?"

"Not that I can think of."

"The family is out of the question?"

"The family is from out in the boondocks. They're not sophisticated enough to give him the care he really requires. They're the first to say so."

"Let's see what we can do to get him into Bart's."

The Committee

When their hectic schedules allow, Lin and Randy like to leave work early on Friday afternoons and drive to "the farm." The land on which Randy's father lives and works is really a cattle ranch 125 miles from Houston. The house the couple shares near the hospital is little more to them than a place to sleep during the week. At the farm, they truly feel at home. On the highway between the two, they sink their shoulders into the seats of Randy's sleek Blazer and try to forget that Hermann hospital exists.

One muggy Friday in September the ride seemed particularly long, the road more congested than usual, the Blazer more cramped. It had been a difficult day. Shortly before she left the building Lin was paged by two of her staff nurses, who were uncomfortable with the care being given to one of their patients. The woman was an elderly diabetic who had already lost her eyesight and had had one leg amputated as a result of her disease. She had been in a coma and on a ventilator for several weeks. Her family was divided over whether the ventilation should be turned off. The nurses thought further use of the machine was futile and were angry that the woman's doctor was making no effort to persuade the family to remove the machine.

"Doctors are jerks," one of the nurses said after explaining the situation to Lin. "We're the ones who see the patients twelve hours straight. We really know them. The doctors have it easy. They round a few times a day, then leave. They don't stay and watch the suffering."

Lin was of a mind to agree, but not in the mood to stay and talk. She would approach the doctor in question on Monday, she promised, as she left to meet Randy. First, she would have to face her own difficult weekend. In the back seat of the Blazer during the drive to the farm sat Lieben, Lin's fifteen-year-old Doberman, sprawled listlessly across the leather upholstery and panting in spite of the air-conditioning. In the front seat, by Lin's feet, was a bag with medication and a hypodermic needle that Lin might use by Monday morning to put the dog to sleep.

In recent years, Lieben's strong, muscular body had begun to fall apart. Her kidneys were weak, her heart was failing, her joints ached, her eyesight was poor. For several weeks, Lin and Randy had discussed painless methods of killing the dog. Painless for Lieben, that is. They knew there was no way to make it painless for themselves. It didn't occur to Lin to ask a veterinarian to do this job in her place. Her savvy dog recognized the route to the vet and began to whimper and shake several blocks away. Randy's cowboy father had once told Lin: "Real men shoot their own horses." She felt she owed it to Lieben to put her nursing training to honorable use and give the injection herself.

It has been more than a decade since Lin Weeks worked at bedside, and in those years she has managed to make the end of life into an intellectual exercise. Death, for all practical purposes, has become a policy question. One of her goals is to codify and streamline the decision-making process at the end of life, and her doctoral thesis includes a checklist doctors can use to explain what they intend when they make a patient DNR. Using her list, death becomes as simple as deciding to give or to withhold any combination of the following: (1) antiarrhythmic drugs; (2) vasoactive drugs; (3) endotracheal intubation; (4) mechanical ventilation; (5) antibiotics; (6) dialysis; (7) blood or blood products; (8) hyperalimentation; (9) tube feeding; (10) cardiac defribrillation; (11) admission to intensive care unit; (12) chemotherapy; (13) invasive monitoring; (14) radiological diagnostics.

Her detachment was hard won. When she first chose nursing as a career, it was because she wanted to become involved and committed, and she was particularly attracted to the drama of the intensive care unit. She took pride in her impatience with authority and bureaucracy, and as early as her first week of nursing school she was nearly expelled for breaking dormitory regulations. Within the first month she was given a reprimand for attempting to correct the staff doctors. She saw it as her job to challenge the rules.

Each year, however, she became drained by the energy required to wrestle with the system and simultaneously care deeply about every patient. Without planning to do so, she drifted into administrative work, directing other nurses and developing her own rules of patient care. She wrote a book about cardiovascular nursing, and she read hundreds of others about management theory, hoping that they would teach her to avoid being the type of administrator she had always despised. She lost none of her skepticism of authority, but she did decide that rules per se were not bad, only bad rules were bad. Rules that were thoughtful and wise could potentially solve problems. So she set out in search of reasonable rules.

This transformation, as it were, was completed the season that her mother fell ill. From Christmas Eve through New Year's Day, Lin and her family battled with the doctor in charge, who refused to remove her mother's ventilator. Each futile argument made Lin feel that she had betrayed her mother by keeping her on a machine that provided maintenance but no cure. She knew her mother's wishes, though they were never put in writing, but for eight days she could not have those wishes carried out. The solution came when Randy educated the doctor about the Texas Natural Death Act, which says that when a doctor cannot honor a patient's wishes, the patient must be transferred to the care of another doctor who is willing to do what the patient asks.

The ventilator was turned off, and Lin was impressed anew at the power of legislation. A Living Will could have solved the problem; a statute book from Randy's office did solve the problem; legalities work where emotion does not.

Because of the way her mother died, Lin is particularly affected by certain types of cases that come before her committee. Teresa Knepper feels most passionately about preemies, like her son, Matthew, who are at the very start of life. Javier Acevas is torn mostly by youngsters, like his son Paco, who have already suffered through much of their lives. Lin's sensitive spot is for patients like her mother, who have lived relatively long lives and want to die in dignity and peace.

These patients at the end of life raise some of the most controversial questions of medical ethics. They also raise the most common ones. In 1988, 11.4 percent of Americans, nearly 27 million people, were over the age of sixty-five, a number that is expected to double by the year 2035. Already there is not enough money to pay for their health care, a situation that will only become worse. Patients sixty-five and older account for 12 percent of the United States population and 33 percent of all hospital admissions each year. Those hospital stays are extremely expensive and often futile. Of all the money spent on medical care over the course of a person's life, two-thirds of the total is spent in the final two weeks. Nearly one-third of the budget of Medicare is spent on patients with less than one year to live.

Numbers such as these have led a few intrepid individuals to wonder in public whether care for older patients should be limited. During the late 1970s, Colorado governor Richard Lamm suggested that terminal patients have a duty to refuse intensive and expensive medical intervention and to die instead, an opinion that brought outraged response from the press, the public, and health officials nationwide. About a decade later, in 1987, bioethicist Daniel Callahan authored a book titled *Setting Limits: Medical Goals in an Aging Society*, suggesting that health care be rationed to older patients. Callahan, too, generated criticism, but he also sparked thoughtful debate. The idea of limiting care to the elderly was beginning to sound less radical and more inevitable.

The Hermann Ethics Committee tries to keep the economics of care out of their discussion about individual cases. The problem of finances always manages to enter Room 3485, but it is confined, metaphorically, to the back of the room and almost never invited to sit at the conference table. Instead, the debate over care for elderly patients is much the same as the debate over younger patients: "How much is too much?" "Is life in this condition really a life?" Her mother always on her mind, Lin most often opts for death.

She occasionally visits these older patients before the committee meets to discuss their cases. Most committee members never visit the patients, an unofficial practice based partly on time constraints and partly on some members' belief that a mental image of the patient makes it more difficult to form a rational, intellectual conclusion about the case. When the patient is older and the question is whether to withdraw life support, Lin often finds herself at the foot of that patient's bed, paying silent homage to them and to her own past.

It is a practice she almost stopped after seeing Eunice Fence. The ninety-seven-year-old woman had been living in a nursing home for several years, her mind wandering between the past and the present, until Labor Day weekend when she had a severe stroke. She was brought to the Hermann emergency room, where doctors used every available type of technology to revive her. Once she was stabilized, it was discovered that the point where her stomach joined her small intestine was almost completely blocked and she was in danger of starving slowly. The surgical staff suggested an operation to insert a feeding tube directly into the small intestine through which she could be fed.

This recommendation troubled the attending doctor. To perform the operation would be inhumane, said the doctor. To withhold the operation would be manslaughter, said the surgeons. The woman's only relatives, two elderly cousins, could not be located. An Ethics Committee meeting was called.

Less than an hour before that meeting, Lin went to see Mrs. Fence. The woman, draped in a drafty hospital gown, was reduced to a breathing skeleton. Curled in a fetal position on the narrow bed, her eyes were open but unseeing, her skin was bruised and sallow, her fingernails were a deathly gray. The only sign that the woman was aware of her world came whenever she was touched. At even the slightest pressure on her body, she would shriek in either fear or pain, it was impossible to determine which. Lin left the room only a few moments after she had entered.

"Technically she's not comatose or brain dead, not in a persistent vegetative state," Mrs. Fence's doctor told the assembled members.

"They never should have resuscitated her in the first place," said Lin.

"She's alert," said one of the surgeons. "She responds to external stimuli."

"That's not alert," Lin snapped. "She doesn't even know where she is."

"How about responsive?" Randy asked, sensing Lin's hair-trigger emotions and trying to keep the meeting calm. "Will you buy the word 'responsive'?"

"Her only real response is screaming in agony every time she's touched," Lin said. "I accept the argument that withdrawing nutrition, that's probably active euthanasia. But on the other hand, would anyone here want to live a life like that or have someone else, namely all of us, condemn them to live it?"

"The law says we can't make that decision," Randy reminded her.

"It doesn't matter what the law says," snapped Lin. "The law always lags behind."

She said little else during the remainder of the meeting, as a consensus formed in favor of surgically inserting the feeding tube. In the end, in the interest of unity she even lent her signature to the document Randy handed to her: "The patient has an incapacitating condition and, at the present time, is awake and responsive, but unable to express her desires regarding this issue. Thus, it would not be appropriate to withdraw nutritional support. It is recommended that an attempt be made to surgically place a jejunostomy tube to facilitate nutritional support."

Hers was the last signature on the form, and she penned it reluctantly. "This is one of the most troublesome cases I've seen," she told Randy over dinner that evening. "Do I think this is the ethically right thing to do? No. Do I think it was the right decision for the committee to make? I'd have to say yes."

Mrs. Fence conveniently died the next day, before the surgery could be performed.

Nearly all issues of medical ethics center on a single question: What is the purpose of medical care? To Lin, the answer is simple: To make patients healthier, or, at least, to allow them to derive some pleasure from their life. She is impatient and frustrated by care that does not meet the definition, that simply postpones death and prolongs a miserable existence. The role of her committee, she believes, is to help limit such futility. Her most frustrating moments are when she fails to apply the brakes to rote medicine; her proudest moments are when she succeeds.

A few days before she left for the farm with Randy and Lieben, she notched one such victory. Walking quickly through a hallway on her way to a meeting, she overheard a sentence spoken in a harried, aggravated tone: "The Ethics Committee says we have to, that's why." Checking her watch she headed in the direction of the voice and found two residents discussing a failing patient. The elderly woman had suffered a heart attack several weeks earlier and lapsed into a coma. In recent days she had been stable, not getting better but not getting worse. Her family asked that she be made DNR, and her doctors agreed. Very early that morning, however, she had taken a sharp turn for the worse and the resident on call had made arrangements for a transfer to the ICU. A second resident questioned that decision, wondering whether it might not be more humane to simply allow the woman to die in a private room surrounded by her family.

"Why send a hopeless case back to the ICU?" he asked.

"Because the Ethics Committee says we have to, that's why," came the reply.

Lin approached the adversaries and introduced herself. "Why are you sending her to the ICU?" she asked.

"Because it would be unethical not to."

"What do you mean by unethical?"

"It would be withholding legitimate care."

"She's DNR, isn't she?"

"That's different. That's only if she arrests."

"Is she Supportive Protocol One or Two?"

The resident squinted in confusion for a moment, then began to thumb through the chart he had been holding tightly in his hands.

"Two," he said when he found the answer.

"That means 'No extraordinary measures,' " responded Lin in her best schoolteacher tone. "What would they do for her in the ICU?"

The second resident began to recite the number of machines and procedures that could be used in the ICU but not on the general medical floor. He ticked off each one on his fingers as he spoke. He soon ran out of hands.

"Will any of that cure her?" Lin asked, interrupting the list.

Both young men shook their heads.

"Will it make her more comfortable?"

"Hardly."

"What will it do?"

"Keep her alive. I thought that's what we're here for," came the sarcastic reply.

"For how long?" Lin shot back.

"Not long."

"Then what's the point?"

The resident called his supervising doctor who agreed with Lin's argument. The transfer to the ICU was canceled and the woman died later that afternoon in a quiet, private room.

Lin thought of that exchange as she looked out the window of Randy's Blazer, watching as the city became suburbs and then country. She thought, too, of the diabetic amputee in a coma back at Hermann whose doctor would not persuade the family to withdraw the ventilator. She thought about Lieben, who used to love the farm, especially the hours spent chasing birds, carrying them back like trophies and depositing them at Lin's feet. Not that she equated the fate of a human being with that of a dog, but both, she thought, deserved simple kindness and respect. So much about death, the dignity of death, depends on who is nearby when it takes place. What if she were not passing by when one woman was being transferred to the ICU? What if another woman had a different doctor, one not as uncomfortable removing ventilator support? What if she weren't there to fight for her mother? What if Lieben belonged to someone else?

Saturday morning, Lieben tried to catch a bird. Spotting it through cloudy eyes she struggled to her feet and began to run, as best as she could, in the direction of the fluttering. But her body failed her, and she managed to move only a few feet, dragging her useless rear legs behind her.

Saturday night, Lin and Randy sat on the floor with their dog for a very long time, stroking her ears, nose, and paws, talking to her softly about the good times that were now over. Eventually, Lin filled the two syringes she brought from the hospital. One contained potassium chloride, the other, succinyl chlorate, both in lethal doses. Her hand froze for a moment just before the tip of the needle touched the dog's mottled skin. She was certain that what she was doing was right, but it was so hard, much harder than she expected. Then, with Randy's help, she gave two quick injections straight into the vein. Lieben twitched slightly, but did not cry. She looked up at Lin with a questioning gaze, making Lin wonder if it was too late to change her mind and save the crippled animal. She didn't try. She forced herself to watch as Lieben's eyes drooped closed, and her breathing gradually stopped.

On Monday morning, Lin stopped in to see the diabetic woman and the less-than-persuasive doctor and learned that the ventilator had in fact been removed over the weekend at the request of the family. The patient, to everyone's surprise, kept breathing without the machine. her respiration was weak and would eventually stop, but her death would take longer than her doctors and family had expected.

The doctor began to vacillate and raised the possibility of putting his patient back on the ventilator.

"This is playing God," he told Lin. "I don't feel comfortable with that, the magnitude of that. You make the policies, but I'm the one who actually has to do it. You can't possibly understand how that feels."

Lin looked at him. Their eyes locked. He seemed to relax.

"Yes, I can," she said.

The doctor looked away. "Thank you," he said.

The woman died shortly thereafter. Several weeks later the doctor received a note from her children, thanking him for helping them make such a difficult choice.

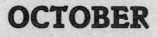

OCTOBER

Patrick

Patrick was not in a good mood. For most of the day he had refused to talk even to those nurses he liked best and instead sat hunched over his Nintendo joystick, finding some sort of comfort in the electronic movement on the television screen. When Javier entered, Patrick, at first, did not even look in his direction. But as soon as the doctor began to speak, the child started to listen, caught by the gravity of the words.

"You know the line is blocked again," Javier said. "We have two choices. We can operate and put in another one, or we can use peripheral IVs."

The answer came back without hesitation, the answer of a frightened child.

"I don't want another operation. You said I wouldn't have another operation."

"You know what will happen with the IVs?" Javier asked.

Patrick nodded, but Javier knew that the child's understanding went only so far. What Patrick understood was that, as each IV became clogged, he would be poked with needles until another site could be found. He would lose weight and feel weak because not enough nutrition could be dripped through the smaller, less efficient tubes. Patrick knew he would hate this, but he also knew he would hate surgery more. That would mean the operating room and a tube down his throat, and disorienting drugs and a lot of pain. He never wanted to go through that again.

What Patrick didn't really understand was that eventually the reliance on peripheral IVs would kill him. If by some miracle enough usable sites could be found in which to stick the IV needles, then he would starve slowly, because the number of calories he needed to sustain even his tiny body could not fit through the tube in the course of the day. If, as was more likely, no more sites could be found, he would starve more rapidly, since he would have no source of calories whatsoever.

For a moment, Javier considered explaining all this to Patrick, but decided instead to keep silent. It was true that by rejecting the surgery Patrick was ultimately choosing death. But by choosing the surgery he would be effectively choosing death, as well, and Javier did not have the heart to explain that quite yet. Instead he inscribed a note in the overflowing chart and left the hospital for the night.

"I have talked with Patrick very openly about this, and *he* has chosen to continue with our present plans and has accepted the need to use peripheral IVs once this line is permanently obstructed," he wrote. "Would continue Vancox 7–10 days in hospital and then plan for discharge."

Two days later the central line failed completely, and Plan B was begun. The insertion of IV lines is usually left to the nurses, but Javier inserted Patrick's first line himself. He calmed the boy with 3 milligrams of morphine, gave a quick jab to the left forearm with a sharp needle, then threaded the thin plastic catheter through the needle. It was the only time in the months before or after that the insertion took only one try.

Patrick's decision was torture for those who loved

him. Every day, sometimes several times a day, the search began for a piece of vein that would accept the thin plastic tube. If Kay was in the building, then Patrick demanded that she alone insert the IV, and her stomach burned with each attempt. The procedure should have taken less than five minutes, but with Patrick it could take hours. He would always insist on holding someone's hand as he watched Kay pierce his skin, five, six, seven times. He would suggest spots that she might try, and sometimes they would argue over whether a particular vein would work.

"Patrick, can I please start here?" Kay would ask.

"No. I want you to try here."

"But, Patrick, I don't think that will work."

"Try it."

"Okay, I'll try it, but if it doesn't work, then I get to pick."

"I know you can do it," Patrick would say.

"Please," Kay would think, "don't have that kind of faith in me."

As the days passed, Patrick's IV ended up in ever stranger parts of his body—his thumbs, his knuckles, his biceps. In fact, the only place he declared off limits was the crease inside his elbows because he wanted to be able to bend his arms. Each day he became steadily weaker, sleeping nearly all day and abandoning Nintendo almost completely. He rarely trotted out to visit the nurses' station, choosing instead to stay curled in his bed with his back facing the door. For a little while, he was encouraged to eat solid foods, in the hope that he would receive some additional calories, but the resulting cramps and diarrhea were so painful that he stopped.

Several times each day someone would test his central line to see if it had cleared. Once or twice there seemed to be reason for hope, but when Javier acted on the glimmer of good news and tried to drip ampho through the line, it blocked again. Without the ampho, the ever-present bacteria that lived within Patrick gathered strength, and Javier wondered whether starvation or infection would claim the child first. Javier's twice daily visits to Patrick's bedside became more difficult, and Javier's resolve began to weaken.

"No fever yet," he wrote in the chart one evening, a week after Patrick was admitted to Hermann. "I would expect that the candidemia will worsen in the coming days. We will again discuss the surgical 'alternative.' "

Landon

Elsewhere in the country, it was autumn. But in Houston, the thermometer still looked like summer. Early fall is arguably the worst time of year in Houston. Reporters on the national news have put on sweaters. Sports pages of the local newspaper list football scores. Displays in the produce section of the grocery store include pumpkins. Body and mind are ready for a cool front, a break, a relief. But the weather doesn't play along. It is as numbing and as disheartening as a snowstorm in April after a long New England winter.

It had been a particularly long summer at Hermann Hospital. The Ethics Committee had seen its busiest stretch in memory: Patrick Dismuke; Taylor Poarch; Armando Dimas; Mr. Hardy; Mrs. Fence; Dexter Advani; an AIDS patient whose lover wanted treatment continued and whose mother did not (the ventilator was removed); a mentally retarded, severely handicapped girl who needed risky, expensive, experimental surgery (it was not done). In all, there were twelve hard cases in five long months. Everyone on the committee was tired.

If the Hermann Ethics Committee was looking for a break, they didn't get one. The temperature remained near the 90s, and the committee was called to hear another case. It was a case that most members would describe as their toughest ever. When it was over, nearly everyone involved wondered whether they had made the wrong choice.

Days before she would appear at this most difficult of committee meetings, a happily pregnant woman named Claire Sparks spent an afternoon puttering in her unborn baby's nursery. Her baby shower had been the day before, and there were dozens of presents to be put away. Nearly everything was in the pattern she had selected, called Teddy Beddy Bear, which had a light brown bear wearing pastel pajamas and a nightcap. She put the dust ruffle, comforter, and sheets on the crib, filled the diaper bag, put the tiny baby clothes in the dresser drawers, and looked happily around the room.

Claire and her husband, Kenny, don't have much by some people's standards, but they take meticulous care of what they have. Their home is a three-bedroom, two-bathroom Fleetwood trailer, 16 feet wide and 76 feet long, painted brown and cream on the outside. They own it outright, and they also own the land on which it sits—a tree-filled parcel near the end of a sparsely populated dirt road in Dayton, sixty miles east of Houston. They decided on a movable home because they never know when Kenny's job as an oil refinery construction worker might take him to another place. And they chose this particular plot of land because it would be a perfect place for a little boy to play.

The Sparkses had been trying for seven years to have the baby that would complete that picture. The last of an endless parade of doctors suggested that Claire have surgery, an ovarian wedge resection, where a slice of the organ is removed and the remainder is sewn back together. That procedure, combined with powerful drugs to induce ovulation, resulted in something Claire had become convinced she would never see—a positive pink circle on her home pregnancy test.

By October, she was six months pregnant, and certain she was going to have a boy. The sonogram she'd had three months earlier was unclear, but she was certain, nonetheless. Ever since she saw her baby's shadowy picture on the ultrasound screen, she sensed he was a boy and she planned to name him Landon, after Michael Landon, her favorite actor.

Kenny was thrilled at the idea of a son. Like every parent everywhere, he wanted the baby to have what he never had, and for Landon that would mean a challenging job where he could sit at a desk and wear a tie. For Kenny, whose hands were rough and dingy from building and repairing the insides of refinery tanks and whose clothes were sometimes so greasy that Claire wouldn't wash them in her own machine but would take them instead to the coin laundry, a white shirt and a tie were the definition of success.

As dinnertime approached on that October Sunday, Claire clicked off the light in the bear-filled baby's room and went to the kitchen to prepare a beef and macaroni casserole. It was almost finished when Kenny got home from work. With a sigh of exhaustion he eased himself onto the worn couch just outside the kitchen. Claire wiped her hands on a dishtowel and walked from the kitchen into the den to welcome him home.

That was when she felt something warm and wet on her leg. At first she wondered if her amniotic sac had broken. Or maybe her bladder had failed her, with the pressure of the baby and all. Embarrassed, she headed for the bathroom hoping Kenny wouldn't notice. By the time she reached the toilet, there was blood everywhere, and she heard herself screaming her husband's name. Kenny came running. His first thought was that his bathroom looked like a murder scene.

Kenny carried his wife to the car and careened along Highway I-10 to the nearest community hospital, making the twenty-five-mile trip in fourteen minutes. He was certain that his baby was already dead, and he was worried about his wife. He didn't believe someone could lose that amount of blood and survive. Claire, delirious with fear, laughed most of the way to San Jacinto Methodist Hospital in Baytown. They were like a twosome from a Keystone Cops comedy, she thought, weaving through traffic and honking and flailing at any cars that came in their way.

They both talked nonstop, each trying to keep the other calm.

"We've tried for so long to have a baby, and now I've messed this up," Claire said. "I know it's something I did, it's my fault."

"It's not your fault, you did everything the doctor said," Kenny responded. He didn't say what he was really thinking: "Forget the baby. I don't want *you* to die."

Near the end of the ride they crossed paths with a policeman, who signaled them to pull onto the shoulder of the highway. When the man was within shouting distance, Kenny screamed out an abridged version of their situation. The officer ran back to his car, turned on his lights and siren, and leap-frogged with Kenny's car from one intersection to the next, stopping the opposing traffic as Kenny and Claire passed.

The officer also radioed ahead to the hospital, and when the Sparkses arrived, there was a wheelchair waiting.

"You're the one having a baby?" the attendant asked. Obviously the police officer had misunderstood.

"No," sobbed Claire, "I'm not. I'm losing a baby."

The attendant shoved her into the chair and raced

down the hall, running so fast that Kenny lost track of which way they went. He didn't have to ask directions; he simply followed the trail of Claire's blood to the obstetrics area.

By the time he arrived, Claire had been strapped to a fetal monitor, and the doctor on duty had found the baby's heartbeat.

"He's still alive?" Kenny asked.

"He is so far," came the reply.

Fifteen minutes later, Claire was unconscious in a nearby operating room undergoing an emergency cesarean section. Kenny was not allowed to be with her, and he paced alone in the waiting room. The baby was born at 9:48 in the evening, ten weeks early, weighing only 3 pounds and 5 ounces. As soon as he arrived, the obstetrician, Dr. Dan Lucius, handed him off to the on-call pediatrician, Dr. Alton Prihoda, and turned his attention to stabilizing Claire, who had lost a tremendous amount of blood. Both men were slightly shaken. The sleepy Baytown hospital doesn't see a lot of cases as dramatic as this one.

The anesthesia had not fully worn off when a nurse put her hand on Claire's arm and told her, "You have a little boy."

"Is he dead?" Claire asked.

"No, but a helicopter is coming to take him to Hermann Hospital."

Moments later, the obstetrician walked in and asked, "What did you name your little girl?"

"I don't have a little girl, I have a little boy," Claire said.

"No, honey, you have a little girl," the doctor said, in the voice of one who is used to talking to patients still confused by anesthesia.

So Claire decided the nurse was wrong, the doctor

was right, and the baby was a girl. "Okay, if she's a girl, her name is Kendy," she said.

The doctor left and returned five minutes later. His tone of voice had changed. "Claire, honey, you're right, it's a little boy. I guess I didn't check."

"I knew he was a boy," she said. "His name is Landon."

It was only the first of many times that Claire and Kenny Sparks would be confused by contradictory information from their doctors.

Before the helicopter arrived, Kenny was allowed to spend time with Landon. A nurse ushered him into the nursery where his son slept in a Plexiglas-walled isolette wearing only a diaper. Told he could look but not touch, Kenny immediately knew there was something wrong. He didn't know a lot about babies and he hadn't spent much time with them, but he was certain that Landon didn't look like a baby should. There was a startling mass on his back that was tough for Kenny to look at, and it took him a while to realize that what he was seeing was Landon's spinal cord showing through his nearly transparent skin. A red, raw bump covered the cord, but not very well.

A nurse hovered nearby, but Kenny didn't ask any questions. He knew there was something very wrong with his baby, and he knew, too, that he would learn what it was in due time. Whatever the problem, he simply assumed it would kill the boy, so his first concern would have to be his wife. He lingered at the bassinet several minutes more until someone he had never seen before announced that they were taking the baby away, first to his mother's room and then to the waiting LifeFlight helicopter. Kenny followed the isolette as it was wheeled down the hall to Claire's bedside where, through the haze of sedation, she reached into the walled crib, stroked the tiny baby's head and told him she loved him. Landon was facing toward her, and she didn't even notice the gap in his back.

The visit lasted only a moment, and the isolette was wheeled away again. Minutes later, the thwapping sounds of a helicopter broke the silence.

Patrick

Dr. Richard Andrassy was not the least bit surprised when Javier arrived at his office to discuss, yet again, the option of operating on Patrick. It was a conversation he had been hoping to avoid. He would have preferred that Javier decide simply to keep Patrick comfortable, giving him fluids and painkillers to ease his inevitable death. "If I were Patrick," Dr. Andrassy thought, "that's what I would want. I would choose to die before I went through all those painful operations, intubations, tubes, and all that, knowing full well that I'll never be better. If I had to live with that much pain until I died," he thought, "I would much rather die."

Javier didn't feel that way. As usual, he was drawn to the surgeon's cluttered quarters by emotion rather than reason. His well-trained brain knew that further surgery would be essentially useless, but his stubborn streak, his compassion, his belief that he could defy the odds, in short, everything that led him into this profession in the first place, kept pushing him to try just one last time.

This time, the answer Javier received from Dr. Andrassy was "yes." A highly qualified yes, but a yes all the same. "We could try again," he said. "I would be willing to do that.

"We would have a very high mortality risk," he added, stopping short of explicitly adding what both men understood: Maybe it would be better for everyone involved if Patrick simply died on the operating table.

Immediately after leaving Dr. Andrassy's office, Javier tried to find Oria Dismuke to ask permission to operate on her son. It had been weeks since he had spoken with her, and he was not surprised that she was not in Patrick's room, at her home, or behind the hamburger grill at work. In recent months she had been nearly impossible to find. She failed to return phone calls or keep appointments.

"She has a new man, and that's all she has time for," Sally said bitterly.

Oria had a different view. She wasn't being irresponsible. In fact, it took a tremendous amount of concentration and effort to avoid Javier and Sally. "I know what they want to tell me," she said. "They want to tell me my boy is gonna die. They keep saying we have to talk about it, about that he's gonna die. I know he's gonna die. I don't want to talk about it. He don't want to talk about it. Why do they keep making us talk? There are lots of nights I've done cried, but I'm not gonna cry in front of them."

To avoid these dreaded conversations, Oria began visiting during hours when she knew, through years of experience with hospital schedules, that Javier would not be around. Once she saw him in the cafeteria when she was on duty, and she hid behind a stainless steel cart until he went away.

She was no easier to locate this October afternoon when Javier sought permission for Patrick's surgery. So rather than speak to the mother, Javier spoke again to the child. This time it was as blunt a conversation as it is possible to have with a sixteen-year-old boy.

"Patrick," he said, "I don't have anything else to offer. I don't know what else we can do. We have two al-

ternatives: one, peripheral IVs, knowing that they don't
last long, knowing that you will get very malnourished,
very weak; two, another surgery. Surgery is very risky.
You could die. I can't guarantee you will come out of
the surgery with a line because there might not be anyplace to put it. If you do come out with a line, the line
will get infected right away. The infection is still in
your body. We haven't cured it yet. So we may never be
able to use the line. I can't guarantee that you will come
out with no complications either. The chance of that is
very small. There will be complications, and they could
be bad."

Patrick was quiet for several minutes after Javier's
soft and anguished speech. "I don't want the surgery,
but I don't want to die," he said.

"You have two days to decide," Javier said. "If we're
going to do surgery and we wait too long, it becomes
more risky."

Minutes after Javier left the room, Patrick summoned
Kay.

"Close the door," he ordered, and Kay knew it was
serious because Patrick almost never wanted to be behind a closed door.

Once the door was clicked shut and Kay was seated
in a chair by the bed, Patrick repeated his conversation
with Javier. Kay's jaw tightened. She couldn't believe
this boy was facing surgery yet again.

"I have some questions," he said. "I want you to tell
me the truth."

"I always do. What do you want to know?"

"Okay, they're going to put the new line back in the
heart, right?"

"Yes."

"Where will the incision be?"

"They'll have to go back over your old scars. They'll reopen your chest, tip to sternum, and go in that way."

"This is serious?"

"Yes. This is serious."

"Really serious?"

"Really, really serious. I know every other time we told you that, but this is real serious. You might not come back from the operating room. This might be it. We might never see you again."

"I know. I don't want that. But remember last summer, when I tried to eat . . ."

There was silence for a few minutes while both of them thought of the weight he had lost during that failed experiment, of how his eyes seemed to grow bigger when it was really his face that was growing smaller as he slowly began to starve. Suddenly, as if to shake that memory, Patrick began asking another stream of technical questions.

"Will I have to be in the ICU?"

"Yes."

"For how long?"

"I don't know, it depends how well you do."

"Will I have to be on the breathing machine?"

"Yes."

"How long?"

"That depends too."

"Do you think I should have the operation?"

Kay swallowed hard and, at a loss for sage advice, settled for speaking the truth. "I don't know," she said. "I wish I did."

Not long before midnight Patrick called Javier at home. "I think I want to do it," he said. "I'll call my mom and tell her she better talk to you."

The next morning Javier summarized the conversation in Patrick's chart: "Called by Patrick to talk about the surgical option. He acknowledges the risks and potential of death during surgery. He also understands that the line will be contaminated immediately and that there is even the possibility that a central line cannot be placed. He knows that he will likely have complications from the surgery and will go to the PCCU.

"I feel that I do not have *any* other option to improve or better his lifestyle and therefore have offered him to participate very actively in this decision. Which I support.

"I have called Dr. Tom Black and Andrassy to participate in the surgery. This will possibly take place on Thursday."

Word spread quickly through Hermann that another operation was scheduled for Patrick. The number of visitors to his room increased, as did the number of acquaintances who stopped to chat with Javier in the halls. Despite the countless people involved with his patient's care, Javier felt very alone with his decision. Perhaps the only person who felt more alone that day was Patrick.

Landon

Kenny Sparks sat in the peach conference room across from the neonatal nursery, the same room where Fran and Carey Poarch had spent so many hours during Taylor's two months of life. Sitting across from Kenny were three somber doctors, each of whom was there to ask the same question: Did Kenny want them to operate on Landon in order to save the baby's life?

In a haze of exhaustion, Kenny heard their questions, but could not give an answer. It was Tuesday afternoon, and he had been awake since early Sunday morning, unable to sleep and unable to stay in one place. Claire was still recovering from her surgery at the hospital in Baytown, and when Kenny went to visit her there, all he could think about was Landon, tiny and alone at Hermann, and soon he would find himself at the wheel of his car driving the sixty miles to Houston. Yet as soon as he arrived at Landon's crib, he would be torn by thoughts of Claire, distressed and in pain in Baytown, and he would return to the wheel again. He filled the ample tank twice in two days.

Each time he left Hermann, Kenny brought more Polaroid pictures of Landon for Claire. He did so despite the fact that they made her cry when she saw that the baby's legs were almost black because the mass on his back had cut off their circulation. Kenny would start crying, too, and soon he would be off to Hermann again, burning more fuel, taking more pictures, and becoming more exhausted still.

The rare moments that he actually took a pause came during meetings such as this one, when he sank into the cushioned chair that Fran and Carey had come to know so well. Trying to focus on the trio of doctors sitting there with him, he realized they agreed on only one thing: Landon's was one of the most severe cases of spina bifida that they had ever seen.

Between the three of them, the doctors had seen a lot of spina bifida cases. The condition is one of the most common types of birth defects, occurring in two of every 1,000 births, and because Hermann is a referral center for so many smaller hospitals in the region, at least two cases arrive in the nursery every month. The term "spina bifida" is Latin for a spine that is split in two, but that doesn't fully explain what had happened to Landon. Doctors do not know yet the cause of the condition, but they do know that it has its roots during the fourth week after conception, before many women even know they are pregnant. At that time, an embryo is the size of a grain of rice and, in normal embryos, a flat strip of cells down the center begins to fold in on itself and sink into the middle of the organism. As the ends roll toward each other, they form a tube, a process that begins in the middle and works toward each end, much like the closing of a zipper. When everything proceeds as it should, the upper end becomes the brain and the lower end becomes the spinal cord, which is eventually covered with bone, muscle, and skin.

But when Landon was at this crucial stage, everything did not proceed as it should have. Spina bifida occurs when a section of the flat strip of cells is prevented from forming a tube and sinking into the embryo. That in turn means that bone, muscle, and skin can't form around the tube, and the result is a jarring mass like the one on Landon's back. It is called a meningomyelocele, a word Kenny could not remember in those early days despite the countless times it was used by Landon's doctors. "Myelo" means the spinal cord, they would explain, "meninges" refers to the membranes that cover the spinal cord, "cele" is the sac that formed around the cord and the meninges where they protrude out of the unzipped portion on Landon's back.

No one is exactly sure what causes spina bifida. From the moment Landon was born, Claire blamed herself. She was certain she had done something wrong before or during her pregnancy: the fertility drugs, perhaps, or the sessions at the tanning salon before she knew she was pregnant. Her doctors told her not to blame herself, but they could not tell her that her theories were wrong. They simply did not know what caused her son's condition.

Something else they did not know was how the lesion on his back would limit Landon's life. A standard rule of thumb is that location is everything; the higher the lesion sits on the back, the more it limits the baby's future. Each fraction of a millimeter upward increases the chance that the child will need leg braces, be wheelchair-bound, have bowel and bladder problems, or suffer any of the countless other limitations that can come with spina bifida. By this measure, sacral lesions, near the bottom of the spine, are less serious than lumbar lesions, which are at the level of the waist. Landon's lesion began at the lower thoracic spine, in the area of the chest, and gaped 4 centimeters upward toward his neck. It provided no reason for optimism.

The standard procedure for spina bifida babies is a two-pronged surgery. First, the lesion on the back is covered with a fold of skin to make it easier to look at and to prevent potentially fatal infection. Second, a tube, called a shunt, is placed in the skull and down the neck to drain the spinal fluid that tends to build up in the brain. One thing surgery cannot do, however, is fix the damage done by the lesion. The operation would keep Landon alive, but it wouldn't make him better.

All this was first explained to Kenny by Dr. José Garcia, who was the attending physician in the neonatal nursery when Landon was brought to Hermann. With his soft voice, his doughy, gentle face, and his unabashed habit of becoming attached to his patients, José is Sharon Crandell's emotional opposite. Yet both he and Sharon chose neonatology for the same reasons: It is an evolving specialty, a cutting edge specialty, filled with challenging crises that require immediate response.

Kenny's first meeting with José came just a few hours after Landon arrived at Hermann. There was another doctor present at that first conversation, a neurosurgeon, Dr. Hatem Megahed, the same doctor who so vehemently opposed disconnecting Mr. Hardy's ventilator after the man's paralyzing car accident. Together, the two men described the seriousness of Landon's condition to his stunned father. Standing by the baby's bassinet, they carefully uncovered the lesion, lifting the 4×4 square of sterile gauze to reveal the mess beneath.

"What you're looking at, basically, is the covering of the spinal cord," José said, then quickly replaced the gauze.

"Watch his limbs," José continued, staring down at the baby, who was lying on his stomach, groggy but awake. "He can move his arms well but there is no movement in his legs. We haven't seen any sign of function in his lower extremities. No reflexes, no anal sphincter tone. I'm afraid it doesn't look promising."

José paused for a moment, and Dr. Megahed filled
the silence. "He shows no sign of hydrocephalus," or
water on the brain, "which is encouraging," he said,
then went on to explain that Landon would most likely
need a shunt. Imagine the brain as a helium balloon, he
said, floating in a sea of spinal fluid. Normally, the
fluid, which is produced in the skull, flows down into
the spinal cord, then back up into the brain again,
where, in effect, it is recycled. But the lesion is like a
hand pulling gently on the string of the brain/balloon,
lowering it just enough to block the space at the base of
the skull so that the cerebrospinal fluid is trapped. As a
result, the fluid level in the skull continues to rise, eventually compressing the brain and swelling the head. A
shunt bypasses the blockage and gives the fluid someplace to go, he explained. Even if there were no fluid
buildup at the moment, he said, the condition was so
common and the risks were so great that the procedure
was necessary.

The insertion of the shunt, José said, was the second
of two operations that Landon would have within days.
Before that, surgeons would have to close the lesion on
the baby's back. He was careful not to raise Kenny's ex-
pectations, explaining that the wound would not go
away, it would simply look a little better once it was
covered over with a flap of skin. "It's not really plastic
surgery," he said, "because they won't be taking a graft
from someplace else. Instead they'll try to move whatever skin and fascia and muscle over that area to close
it and give it some integrity. They'll take the dura and
pull it together and make a little tube that will let the
spinal fluid flow fairly easily. That's all they'll be able
to do."

It never occurred to José Garcia to present the surgery as a choice, to ask Kenny whether or not he

wanted this operation for Landon. As far as he was concerned, surgery was the only option. Perform this standard procedure, and the baby would almost certainly live. Fail to perform the procedure and the baby would almost certainly die. He knew, of course, that Landon's life would be far from easy, but those long-term problems could be handled as they arose, at a future date and by someone else. The immediate, acute problems were his to solve, and the methods at hand were simple and automatic. That is the role of neonatology—solve the now and hand off the later.

Kenny listened carefully during that first meeting with Doctors Megahed and Garcia and asked many questions. Most of those questions were not about the acute problems that were José Garcia's realm, but were instead about the rest of Landon's life, when the surgery would be over, and he would be back home in his parents' care. Would he walk? Would he talk? Would he be able to go to school? Play catch? Hold a job? Have a family of his own? After scheduling the operation for the following day, José gave Kenny the name of a doctor whose job it was to worry about the long-term rather than the here and now.

Like most neurologists', Dr. Ian Butler's job is to step in when the crisis has passed and the chronic, lifelong care has begun. Later that same day, the tall, redheaded Australian doctor loped into the nursery, looked under the piece of sterile gauze, then began to perform many of the same tests on Landon that José Garcia had performed that morning. First, he stood for a few minutes and simply watched Landon. The baby's legs did not so much as twitch. "If he doesn't move his legs, odds are he can't move his legs," Ian said.

Next, the doctor took a rubber-topped hammer from his pocket in order to tap the baby's joints and test his reflexes. The hammer, the same size as those that internists use on adults, looked massive next to the tiny preemie, but Ian has developed a soft touch. Landon did not respond at all as the doctor gently hit the fleshiest part of his patient's tiny knees. "Not too good, kiddie," Ian said.

Several similar tests followed, none of which drew any response from Landon. His arsenal empty, Ian lingered silently at the baby's side for several minutes, sorting in his mind what he would say to the child's parents. This was one of the most severe cases of spina bifida that Ian Butler had seen during his twenty-five years of practice, and the more he thought about it, the stronger his feeling became that Kenny and Claire were being railroaded. Surgery to insert a shunt and close the lesion would probably prolong the baby's life, but he wondered whether that really was the greater good. He had treated countless patients whose bodies and lives were scarred by spina bifida, and while many led happy, nearly normal lives, others merely existed. It was impossible, he realized, to explain to a parent, particularly a brand-new parent, how completely this condition would change their world. But he felt he had a responsibility to try, and he felt Claire and Kenny had a right to reject the planned surgery if they felt letting Landon die would be more humane than helping him to live.

"Very high lesion at mid-thoracic level," he wrote in the chart. "I would give parents option for conservative treatment given the severity of the lesion."

So Kenny found himself in the conference room yet again, this time with Ian Butler. José Garcia had sat there hours before and talked about the next few days. Now Ian talked about the coming years. He explained that Landon would never walk or sit, and that he probably would never speak or hear. His vision might well be impaired. He might have limited use of his hands. He might have severe mental limitations that would not be known for many years.

"I just think you should know there is another option," he told a stunned and silent Kenny. "In these very severe kiddies when there is really no possibility of walking or bladder or bowel control, there is another option of quote unquote 'letting nature take its course.'

"The future management of a kiddie like this, given the number of systems involved, is very complicated. Orthopedists, urologists, neurologists, gastroenterologists, pulmonologists. I may have left out an 'ologist.

"It's very difficult, once you start, to stop. Where do you stop? Do you stop? Do you just fix the back? Do you fix the head? Put a shunt in? Do a brain decompression? If the spine is not straight, do you do scoliosis surgery? At one time there was a lot of bladder work done, now they catheterize the bladder. Then there are hips to be fixed, tendons to be transplanted. Once you start it is very difficult to stop. You should think about whether you want to start and if you want to stop. You can say, 'Look, we're going to fix the back to make nursing easier, but if the child develops hydrocephalus, we're going to make another set of decisions as to whether or not to pursue that.' You need to be aware this is a lifelong medical commitment."

He paused, waiting for questions from Kenny. There were none, and he continued.

"I can't predict what's going to happen. No one can. Just because you don't do anything doesn't mean your child will die of the complications of the disease. He may be a very highly resistant customer and survive his meningitis and ventriculitis and all those sorts of things. You have to understand that that can happen, and he could survive even if you don't do the surgery. We've had cases like that, and then they end up with a big head at three or four from all the fluid that builds up. Their head's so big they can't carry it around."

The next morning José brought Kenny the consent forms for the surgery that was scheduled hours later. Kenny refused to sign. "Dr. Butler said we shouldn't have the operation," he said.

Troubled and enraged, José tracked down Ian Butler, who summarized what he had told the young father the afternoon before.

"Are you serious?" was the first thing José could think to say.

"Quite serious," Ian said. "I think they should have a choice."

"This is the standard of care, it's the way it's done," José protested.

"It wasn't the standard of care until five years ago, when the Baby Doe case sent everyone running for cover," answered Ian. "I'm not saying we should kill any baby with a problem. I'm not saying we should kill this baby or even let him die. I'm saying the parents should know what's coming and make a choice, and part of that choice should be the option of not doing anything at all."

"You want to withhold treatment based not on a lethal lesion, because this lesion alone won't kill him, but based on the quality of life the baby is going to have if it survives?" José asked. "Even if that weren't illegal— and I think it probably is—I don't know if I want to start assuming that right."

"We shouldn't assume that right. The parents should. That's my point."

The increasingly acrimonious discussions left Kenny ricocheting between doctors as he bounced between hospitals. His problem wasn't that he couldn't make a decision. He made a lot of decisions, all of which contradicted the prior ones. When he talked to José Garcia, he saw pain and pleading in the younger doctor's eyes, and he agreed that surgery was the best approach. When he talked to Ian Butler, sometimes moments later, he was struck by the older doctor's calm rationality, and he decided he couldn't possibly subject his son to the hellish existence the neurologist described. The Tuesday surgery was canceled and rescheduled for Wednesday. The doctors kept asking for an answer. Kenny kept changing his mind.

"Okay," he told José, "if this is what we need to do, let's get it done."

Five minutes later, at the other end of the hallway, Ian Butler asked the same question.

"We're not going to do anything," Kenny said.

Kenny's indecision was made worse by the fact that this dilemma was his to solve alone. His family spoke to the doctors with him, as did Claire's family, but all the relatives made it clear that although they would support whatever he decided, they wouldn't tell him what to do. Claire was in no shape to decide anything. The way she copes with pain is to sleep or to cry, and she was all cried out by the morning after Landon's birth, so she spent most of the following two days fast asleep. Escape from her problems was made easier by the pain pills the nurses brought every few hours.

So the choice was Kenny's, and he could not choose. On Wednesday morning, after three days without sleep, he sat slumped in the conference room with his mother, Claire's brother, and Doctors Butler and Garcia and listened yet again to the pros and cons. It was time to make a final choice, the doctors said. The surgery is scheduled for this afternoon.

"Have you thought about whether or not to operate?" José asked.

"Have I thought about anything else, that's the better question. I think I'm leaning against it. I think maybe we should let nature take its course."

José was ready for that answer.

"I think you should know," he said, "that I talked to the hospital's lawyer, and we would probably have to go to court if it comes to that. We would ask them to appoint another guardian for Landon and ask for a court order to do the surgery anyway."

This was news to Ian. "That's nonsense," he said, his mouth set into a tense line.

"Under Texas law a patient has to have a terminal illness to withhold treatment, and this isn't a terminal illness," José said, repeating what Randy Gleason had told him the night before. "If you decide not to operate, we'll have to call the hospital attorney for his opinion. I also think we should call the Ethics Committee."

Kenny was filled with new energy. Instead of slumping in his chair as he had done moments earlier, he sat upright and angry. He had been emotionally paralyzed by the idea of choosing Landon's fate. But the idea that he would not be *allowed* to make that choice made him furious. The uncertainty he had felt in recent days lifted. He was absolutely certain now, and he would not let any hospital change his mind.

"Why are you asking my opinion if you're going to go ahead and operate anyway?" he asked, his voice electric with rage.

José didn't answer, and Kenny lowered his voice to ask one last question, the one nearly every patient asks and every doctor hates to hear.

"What would you do if it were your baby?" he said.

José thought of his own seven-year-old son, whose

photo is the only decoration in his spare office, and said, "I would sign the consent form."

Ian thought of his own three children, grown and healthy, and said, "I would not."

In the end, Kenny asked for one more day. "I have to talk to Claire," he said. "She's his mother, and I can't do this by myself."

The surgery was rescheduled yet again, for Thursday morning, and Kenny drove the numbing route back to San Jacinto Methodist Hospital in Baytown. Claire was asleep, and he sat silently by her bed for nearly an hour until she opened her eyes and tried to focus on his face. He spoke slowly, repeating everything several times to make certain that she understood. He explained what spina bifida is, how serious a case Landon had, and what the different doctors had said. When he finished, they held hands in the dimly lighted room for a while until Claire found a shaky voice for her thoughts.

"Let's not rush into surgery," she said, as tears welled and burned her eyes. "This is going to sound terrible for a mother to say, but I want him to die. It would be best for him. It's not really living if you're just going to lie there all your life and do nothing. They don't even know if he'll come out of the surgery, and then we'll have to do surgery after surgery."

Kenny started to speak, but she interrupted, defending her choice against the opposition she assumed was coming.

"If he lives, that's the way it should be," she said. "But if he dies, I can live with that."

It was nearly midnight when Kenny left Bayton hospital and drove back to Hermann. He wanted to say goodnight to Landon. When he arrived, he found José Garcia sitting at the nurses' station in the center of the room. Kenny nodded hello without stopping to talk and

went directly to Landon's crib. Several minutes later a nurse interrupted. "Dr. Garcia would like to speak to you before you leave," she said.

Kenny approached the desk and saw that the doctor was holding a surgery consent form, rubbing the edge between his thumb and forefinger like a good luck charm.

"If I asked you to sign this right now, would you or wouldn't you?" he asked.

"No," Kenny said, "I wouldn't."

"You realize that means he may die?"

"I realize that."

Kenny thought he saw tears well in José's eyes. The doctor nodded slowly, a sad, tired nod, and left through the swinging metal doors. Kenny left soon afterward and made the hour-long trip home, where he fell into a nightmare-filled sleep.

Patrick

Patrick called Kay at midnight to tell her he didn't think he would be able to sleep. Then he called again at 5 A.M. to say he was right, he hadn't slept at all. Kay really hadn't slept either. "No, you didn't wake me," she told him honestly at the start of each of the calls. "I'll be there in a little while," she said at the end of the second one.

In the three hours between her arrival at the hospital and the time orderlies came to take Patrick to the operating room, Kay sat at the nurses' station, and Patrick sat at her side. They didn't talk much, and when they did, it was little more than nervous chatter. When the phone call finally came at 9 A.M., announcing that a stretcher was being sent for Patrick, Kay thought briefly about hiding him. As was his particular custom, he refused to lie down on the stretcher, but insisted instead on being wheeled away sitting up, yoga style. Kay draped a blanket over his legs and gave him a good-luck kiss, but didn't walk with him to surgery. Richard did, and as the short, somber procession headed toward the elevator, Richard looked back sorrowfully at Kay. Both of them hated the idea of another operation, but they understood Javier's need to give it a try.

"It's easy for me to say I wouldn't do it," Richard

told Kay when they first learned that the surgery had been scheduled. "I'm not the one who has to sign the order that says, 'Let him starve to death.'"

Richard stayed with Patrick once he was inside operating room number 10. The boy wouldn't lie down there, either. Over the years, he had developed a terror of the anesthesia mask, and he would insist that he be put to sleep while he was sitting up. So he was injected with sedatives to calm him enough that he would not struggle when the threatening mask was placed over his face. As he drifted off, the loudspeakers in the operating room, which usually played Dr. Andrassy's favorite classical music, played the rap and rock that Patrick loved. Richard stood by his side until the injection took effect, and Patrick's hand went limp in his own.

After Richard left, the assembled nurses and surgery residents prepared Patrick's unconscious body. They stretched him flat on his back on the operating table and surrounded him with mounds of padding. A foam roll was placed under his shoulders, another cradled his head, his arms lay at his sides on foam pillows, rolled towels were wedged under his knees, and each heel was given its own spongy cushion. His lower body was draped with a metallic warming blanket. His upper body was scrubbed with antiseptic and draped with the deep blue cloths that indicate a sterile area. Only his chest and its montage of scars was exposed.

At that point, Dr. Andrassy entered the room. He prefers to wait until his patients are draped and unconscious before he sees them. It is easier that way to forget that the body on the table, a body he is about to slice, splice, and sew, is a person. As he walked toward Patrick's draped figure, he looked into the spectators' gallery and noticed it was empty. Of all the people who loved Patrick so, not one wanted to come and watch. Dr. Andrassy understood. "They beg me to operate but they can't bear to look," he thought. "They don't want to be here if he dies. They would rather have me come back up and say he died than watch it. I wish I could be someplace else, too."

The operation actually began at 10:48 A.M., nearly two hours after Patrick said good-bye to Kay. In a brutal opening act that belied the delicate procedure to follow, Patrick's rib cage was split open with an electric saw. This is usually the fastest part of any heart operation, but this time it was tedious and slow. The same skin and bone had been cut through so often over the years that it was a dense tangle of scar tissue. Under normal circumstances, the chest wall should simply pull up and away, exposing the heart. Patrick's chest wall was attached to his heart in some places by unyielding scar tissue, and to yank too quickly at the chest wall could rip the heart itself.

As he snipped and burrowed through the bloody thicket, Dr. Andrassy talked constantly, explaining his every motion to the medical students and surgery residents who ringed the operating table. Talking is his way of dissipating the tension.

"He's had so much scarring and fibrosis and all that it's just a mess in here," he said from behind his surgical mask. "It's like chipping through cement to get down to the heart. What worries me in all this digging is that instead of getting into the scar tissue around the heart, we'll get right into the heart. Be prepared for that. I might have to fix the heart."

Dr. Andrassy finally did reach the heart, without catastrophe. With a flourish, he tugged at the old catheter until it slid out into the air. Holding it aloft for a moment before placing it in a sterile dish, he noted the black-red clot still clinging to its tip. "There's our problem," he said, as a nurse took the steel dish from the table and prepared to send it to the lab for a routine culture.

Then he shook his head. "No, that's not really his problem," he said. "His problem is his body is breaking down. The infection leads to changes in permeability, fluids escape from the vessels into the tissue, and little by little the body dies from the inside out. The cells die first, and then the organ dies, and then the body dies."

Dr. Andrassy had hoped to sew the new central line into the opening of the heart where the old one had been. But the clot in the line was matched in size and density by the clots left behind in the heart and, after several unsuccessful attempts, the surgeon reluctantly stitched closed the old entrance point to the left side of the heart and created a new one in the right atrium instead.

"With all the operations he's had and with his lousy nutrition over the years, the heart tissue isn't normal," he explained aloud as he struggled to close the old opening. "Instead of firm tissue, it's like cottage cheese. Cottage cheese won't hold a stitch."

With much effort, Dr. Andrassy secured the new tube in place with a stitch known as a purse-string suture, named because it closes around the line like the neck of a drawstring purse. Such a stitch would hold the line indefinitely, but could be removed with a sharp, deliberate yank on the end that would be exposed to the air. Should this line stop working, there would be no need to cut Patrick open again to remove it. And, there would be no need to bury him with it.

Once the line was secure, Dr. Andrassy stabbed a small
hole in Patrick's right chest wall and eased the new line
from the inside to the outside, sewing it in place exter-
nally with nylon thread. The difficult part was over.
Most of what was left was on the order of housekeep-
ing. Water was poured into the chest cavity, to clean
away the pooling blood, then suctioned out again. A
drainage tube was placed through the chest wall. The
rib cage was remolded and held in place with thin, flexible wire. The surrounding muscle and deep layers of
skin were sewn together again. The entire wound was
closed with a surgical staple gun that lifts and pinches
the skin as it inserts a two-pronged, curved staple. The
sponges were counted and recounted. Thirty had been
used, and thirty had been removed. The needles were
similarly tallied, and all twenty-one were accounted for.
The operation was completed at 1:25 P.M. There were
no complications.

Javier did not attend the operation. Though he often
observes surgery on his patients, he couldn't watch this
one, and he spent much of the two and a half hours with
Jan Van Eys, who just happened to stop by for a cup of
coffee.

Sally Olsen passed the time alone at her desk, shuffling papers and hoping that Patrick would die on the
operating table. That would be the only blessing of surgery, she thought. What a neat, clean way to get him
out of this messy, impossible life.

Kay and Richard busied themselves near the third-
floor nurses' station. Every so often, one of the two
anesthesiologists would leave the OR and give the
waiting staff an update. When the final report came
that all had gone well, those nurses who could be
spared for a few minutes gathered by the elevators

that would bring Patrick from the operating room to the pediatric ICU. When the doors slid open and his tube-draped stretcher appeared, there was a spontaneous round of applause.

"At least he made it this far," Kay said.

The Committee

One controversial surgery was over. Down the hall and around the corner, in Room 3485, the debate about another controversial operation was far from done. Lin Weeks was the first to arrive at the Ethics Committee meeting about Landon Sparks. She had barely settled in at the square conference table when Sharon Crandell entered and took the seat next to her. Teresa Knepper arrived next and sat on the edge of a chair at the far end of the room with the uncomfortable look of someone trying hard to look relaxed.

Dr. Stanley Reiser and Randy Gleason switched chairs twice, trying to find ones with the padding in place. "They don't want better chairs, that encourages longer meetings," Randy said. "The point is to make the gluteus hurt." The joke did nothing to ease the tension.

When Dr. Margo Cox entered, Sharon scowled and busied herself with paperwork to avoid saying hello. Until recently Dr. Cox had worked as a neonatologist at Hermann and she was still a member of the Ethics Committee. She had just started her own private practice, but during her years at Hermann, she and Sharon often clashed over cases just like this, though they never brought their differences to the committee. The tension and periodic flare-ups that resulted from their radically opposite views on almost every subject were draining for them both, and were among the reasons Dr. Cox was relieved to leave Hermann. Neither woman was looking forward to rehashing those differences again today.

Ian Butler sat on one end of the table with Dr. David Oelberg, who would have been on call the night Landon was admitted had he not asked José Garcia to fill in for him. Jan Van Eys, puffy from a head cold, sat on the other side of Ian. José, the last to arrive, sat with his back to the door, across the table from Ian and Dr. Oelberg. He felt decidedly uncomfortable there.

Checking her watch, then glancing at the clock, Lin quickly introduced Doctors Butler, Oelberg, and Garcia and asked José to introduce the case. "Baby Boy Sparks is a neonate, born October twenty-third, three days ago, at approximately eleven P.M.," he said, in a soft, professional monotone. "The mother is a twenty-six-year-old white female. The father is a twenty-seven-year-old white male. This is her first pregnancy. Prenatal history: Mom had a history of infertility, believed to be Stein-Leventhal syndrome. She took Clomid and became pregnant. There was a negative prenatal ultrasound, negative alpha-fetoprotein. The baby was born in San Jacinto Methodist in Baytown. There was rupture of the placenta, a stat C-section. The infant was preterm and presented with a closed meningomyelocele in the middle of his spine. Preterm problems are that of a thirty-two-week preemie: apnea, patent ductus, not significant. During the second day he required mild oxygen therapy, now on room air. Some anemia, hasn't required transfusions. There are contractures of both extremities, club feet. The neurological exam was remarkable for no movement of lower extremities, no sensation in the lower extremeties."

José paused for a moment and drew in a deep breath.

He began to speak, stopped, drew another breath, cleared his throat several times, then tried again.

"Due to the severity of the lesion, the parents were given two approaches," he said. "The surgery approach, which is the aggressive approach, closing the lesion and knowing it will require a shunt and won't change the prognosis. Or the conservative approach, namely, maybe we should consider no approach at this time. Last night the dad felt he could not sign a consent agreement at that time. He said he would like to 'let nature take its course.' He understands that if the sac ruptures, the child may die from meningitis or ventriculitis. Last night, after he left, there was some leakage. There is also some evidence of hydrocephaly. Since there were two different approaches, that's why we called you.

"The issues as I see and would like to present them, well, the parents have asked me not to provide a procedure that may lengthen his life a bit. I don't know if I can do that. And what if we do take that approach? Do we also refuse to treat him for bouts of sepsis, for infection, for necrotizing enterocolitis?"

José asked his questions with his arms outstretched and his palms facing upward, as if he were waiting for someone to place the answer in his hands. Lin began to speak when he was finished, but she offered no wisdom or solutions. Instead, she asked more questions.

"In other words," she said, "our problem here is we asked the parents to choose conservative or aggressive treatment. They chose conservative. Now we need to determine whether we can permit that."

She turned toward José.

"If the lesion is closed, what is his prognosis?" she asked.

"His prognosis is poor."

"And if it isn't closed?"

"Even poorer."

Sharon shook her head. "If it's closed, he won't be able to walk," she said, "and if it isn't closed, he'll get an infection and die."

"He'll get an infection, sure, but only if the lesion continues to leak," José said.

Jan Van Eys gave a wry laugh. "It will most assuredly leak," he said.

Teresa clenched her fist for courage and changed the subject slightly. "What about his mental state? What will he be able to learn or understand?"

"How do you evaluate the mental state of a thirty-six-week preemie?" Sharon said, in a tone that made Teresa sorry she had asked.

Sharon's tone made Margo Cox bristle. "He has hydrocephaly, so that's a clue," she said.

That comment, in turn, so enraged Teresa that she forgot her seconds-old resolution to keep her thoughts to herself. "My son has problems, too, and he's very bright, so that doesn't impress me," she snapped. "He was premature, and they said he would have damage, and he just brought home a hundred on a spelling test."

"May I explain something?" asked Ian, who had not yet spoken. "In all my years I can't remember ever having raised this issue except on this occasion. This is one of the most severe cases of meningomyelocele I have seen. I felt it was important to give the child other options.

"As for his prognosis, it's more complicated than 'He will not walk.' I'm not saying, 'Don't save him because he will not walk.' I'm saying he will not sit. He will have problems with respiration. He will have neurological problems. This is not mild hydrocephalus, this is significant. This child's head is peculiar looking. There's a malformation at the base of the brain. He's starting out with a lack of brain. He'll require endless surgery, closure of the back, shunting of the hydrocephalus. There will be no bladder function, no bowel function. I thought they ought to know that even after going through all that surgery, they may have a child who just lies there. The problem with a little cure is when do you stop?"

"But what you're saying is we shouldn't start anything because of the possibility that one day the parents might want to stop," José responded. "It's not a question of do everything or do nothing. If we close the baby, and he continues to deteriorate, that doesn't mean we can't sit down with the parents and physician and hospital and say, 'Gee, maybe now enough is enough.' Those decisions are always available. Just because we make this decision doesn't mean we can't rethink it."

"I'm not worried about what happens if he gets worse," Ian said. "I'm worried about what happens if he lives, if he stays the same, or bounces along from one easily curable episode to the next. What are we doing to his parents?"

Dr. Oelberg answered. He had been away at a two-day conference when Landon was admitted. October was his month on call in Turner, and this patient technically became his when he returned early that morning. He had not met Kenny yet, but he had seen the baby, and he was leaning toward recommending surgery, not for ethical, legal, or medical reasons, but because he thought operating would eventually be the easier option for the parents.

"If it's the parents you're worrying about, then surgery, in my experience, is the better route," he said. "Families already feel guilty in a situation like this. They're probably imagining everything they might have done to cause the situation in the first place. They'll only compound that guilt more by sitting and letting a baby die. They've come nine months through the waiting process, they've bonded to the baby even before it's born, and then suddenly there's a calamity. It's always met with guilt. They'll entertain the idea of withholding treatment, but in the last analysis almost all of them change their minds."

"Is this really the easier decision for *them*, or is it the easier decision for *you*, for all of us, because we get to walk away?" Dr. Cox asked.

"Yes, it's easier for me, too," Dr. Oelberg answered. "I feel more comfortable saying, 'Go ahead and do the surgery.' If someone wanted to take this to court, and it went to the Supreme Court, I think it could go either way. There are certainly precedents in the courts for that kind of case being found guilty and the parties involved being found guilty. I have one or two other things to do, and I'd rather not go to the Supreme Court."

"Exactly," Sharon said. "The standard, accepted care for this condition in this community is to close the lesion immediately, and you're deciding to abandon the standard of care because of what his life will be like, so you're making a decision based on handicap."

"The standard of care is irrelevant," Margo Cox said, "because you don't usually see anything like this. This case isn't standard."

"It shouldn't matter how severe the lesion or what we predict for his quality of life," José said. "Hospital policy and state law allow us to abandon treatment for a terminal infant who would die anyway. This is a nonterminal infant. The surgery isn't postponing death, it's lengthening life."

"That's where I have trouble with this," said Dr. Jim Grotta, a neurologist who was about to leave on a year-long sabbatical. "We spend so much time establishing guidelines. Well, does it fall within the purview of those guidelines for us to withhold care because we think the child will grow up retarded?"

"I think we've done it before," Dr. Cox said. "We can't decide this based on what we think the newspapers are going to say, or even what the courts may decide. Our decision has to be about what's ethical. Maybe the law and the guidelines and the standard of care are all wrong."

"Can I jump in here?" Randy asked, and everyone at the table turned in his direction. "I want to say two things. First, the guidelines do not require only a terminal illness in order to withhold care. They apply in the event of (1) permanent unconsciousness, (2) terminal illness, (3) incurable incapacitating illness where further treatment will not reverse the underlying disease process. So I don't think your hands are tied with respect to what the policy says. But I do warn you, and I warn you every strongly, somebody will probably take this to Child Protective Services if the parents stick to their decision."

Dr. Van Eys frowned. "I would hope we could keep this from reaching overzealous eyes," he said quietly.

In the silence that followed there was much shuffling of papers and glancing at watches. Everyone had had his or her say, and everyone was made uncomfortable by the sharp words and the difficult decision.

"I guess it's time we meet the parents," Lin announced, sliding her chair away from the table, then walking toward the closed conference room door. Claire and Kenny, looking tired and pale, were waiting in the hallway. Lin had assumed they were much farther away than that, and sped through the committee's decision in her mind, wondering what they might have overheard. "We have to be more careful about where the parents wait," she thought, as Kenny pushed a wheelchair-bound Claire into the room. Claire's mother followed close behind.

The young parents had absolutely no idea why they were in this bright, crowded room. They knew this was the Hermann Hospital Ethics Committee, but no one had told them—or, at least, they didn't remember being told—what that committee was going to do. As Kenny parked Claire's wheelchair in the only empty space at the table, next to Dr. José Garcia of all people, Claire felt as if she were onstage. She had the starring role, but no one had given her the script.

Less than an hour earlier, Claire had seen Landon for the first time since the night he was born. She had been released from San Jacinto Methodist Hospital three hours earlier, specifically for this meeting. Her departure had been almost like a party, and the nurses had presented her with a bathrobe, a car seat, a photo album, a baby blanket, and a tiny T-shirt that said, "I was born at San Jacinto Methodist Hospital." Not until she and Kenny had waved good-bye to the hospital staff and were driving toward Hermann did the new reality of their life overwhelm her.

"Are they going to try to talk us into surgery again?" she asked Kenny.

"Probably," he answered. "They said they would take us to court."

"He's our baby. We have to decide what's best," Claire said.

"Hell if I know what's best," said Kenny, and they drove the rest of the way in grief-filled silence.

When they arrived at Hermann, Kenny found an attendant with a wheelchair, explained that Claire was too weak to walk, and insisted that his wife sit in the chair during her visit with Landon. It wasn't her *physical* strength that worried him, but he didn't mention that. She agreed to the wheelchair, but then changed her mind. So they left the chair at the nursery door, and Claire walked shakily toward Landon's crib. The closer she came, the tighter she held on to Kenny's hand, trembling partly from weakness, but mostly from fear. "Landon, this is your mother," Kenny said to the sleeping baby. "Claire, this is your son."

She was relieved that there was a patch over the lesion and, unlike Kenny, she didn't ask the nurses to remove it. She had been afraid to look at her baby's back, terrified by dreams that the awful gaping hole went straight through him. She reached down very slowly and ran her finger across Landon's shoulders, which shrugged in reflex. "Hello, Landon, hello baby, I'm your mom." With slightly more confidence, she started to stroke his arm, but the IV got in the way. She rubbed his head. She put her finger in the baby's palm and smiled as his hand closed around it.

As Claire stood silently holding her son's hand, the head nurse walked over and explained that the lesion had begun to leak spinal fluid several hours earlier and was now in imminent danger of infection. It was no longer a question of waiting to see what would happen; it had already happened, and now they had to decide what to do.

Kenny and Claire simply looked at each other. They didn't say a word, but they knew they had finally reached a firm decision. They turned back toward the door where Claire eased gratefully into her wheelchair, allowing Kenny to push her toward the room where the Ethics Committee was waiting.

"Just tell us how you feel," said the woman with short blond hair who had met them at the door and who seemed to be in charge. Kenny stood up, not certain at first what he was going to say. As soon as he began to speak, he knew it would be a while before he would stop. He suddenly had so much to say and his thoughts were tumbling out in no logical order. "Tell us how you feel," the woman asked. In the past three days he had felt every imaginable emotion, and now he was trying to explain them all.

"We'd like to see him grow, to lead as normal a life as we possibly can make it," he said. "He's our first baby, we love him. There's no doubt about that. If he makes it through, he's going to get the best care anybody can give him. We want what's best for him, but we don't know what that is. We can't decide. I don't know how to take four or five opinions and then decide whether my son lives or dies.

"The thing on his back, I feel like it's something God put there. Some people say it's better to have it fixed now. Some people say the surgery will kill him, or his life won't be worth living, or he'll need surgery forever. How do you make the right decision? I don't think there is any right decision. It's just something my wife and I are going to have to live with.

"I don't mean to keep saying 'I' think. I mean *we* think, but she's been in the hospital so it's been me up to now, so I got used to talking that way, but it's me and her. We're both making these decisions.

"Nobody's ever going to know how much we love that baby boy. Today's the first day she's really seen him. He's something me and her wanted for six, seven years. We had docs saying we couldn't. In a sense, this is already our little miracle. If it turns out good or bad, we're going to accept it."

At several points in the soliloquy, Lin began to interrupt with a question, but she caught herself each time. As Kenny's words flowed, they were mesmerizing, and the roomful of sophisticated, hardened professionals simply sat and stared. The parents sitting before them were swollen with grief. They looked almost as if they were a teardrop away from turning liquid and spilling under the table. Everything ran together, his words, her tears, the sodden glances they gave each other the few times Kenny paused for a breath.

Javier arrived late, just as Kenny began to speak. As he listened, he thought of Patrick, of his own decision to perform another kind of operation and of his own doubts as to whether he had made the better choice. Was he doing this for himself or for Patrick? Was the committee thinking of these parents? Were they able to communicate with these parents? Or were they hearing this case because it had raised sticky legal questions in the guise of medical ethics?

Margo Cox was thinking of her brother, four years older than she and living across the country in a group home for retarded, disabled adults. Her thoughts were not of the operation, but of the years after the operation. "We as physicians tend to see a child's survival as a good thing, and we send this devastated child home to a family, a child who can never feed himself, who will always need twenty-four-hour care, and say, 'It's your problem now,' " she thought to herself. "When my parents die, it's going to be a disaster. We're going to have to bring him here. I'm many steps ahead of this poor couple. I'm many steps ahead of most of the people in this room. I've seen a mother who never has a moment when she isn't responsible. I've seen a father without a son. It's better not to have a son than to lose him, and it's better to lose him to death than to have him as a constant burden. It's not that I think all defective children shouldn't live, it's just that I think parents, not courts and committees, should be the ones to decide, and in order to decide they have to know what's in their future."

Teresa, as always, was thinking of Matthew. She was remembering the anguish she felt in the days after he was born, when she couldn't stop crying, and she asked the doctors to explain her baby's conditions over and over again because she couldn't concentrate long enough to remember anything they said. She didn't bathe for a week, and she didn't sleep for nearly that long. She had vivid fantasies about driving her car off the road and into a tree.

Like Dr. Cox, she was imagining what this family faced over the next few years. Unlike Dr. Cox, she believed they should consent to the surgery. She imagined the advice she might give Claire and Kenny: "Every time you look at your baby," she thought, "you'll think, 'He's never going to ride a bicycle, he's probably never going to walk.' You think of all the things that he's not going to be able to do. There are going to be days when all you can do is cry. Your medical bills are going to drive you to the poorhouse. People who were your friends before are not going to be your friends now because they're going to blame this on you. They're going to tell you that you made the wrong decision and that he'd be better off dead. You're going to have to live with all the stuff that people are going to tell you. Then he'll get as old as Matthew, and you'll start to think, 'Hey, maybe it's going to be all right after all.'

"I have to be real careful talking to people," she continued silently. "I can tell them there's hope, and then they may get the baby home and the day-to-day reality will hit them, and they'll think about me and say, 'What did she do to me?' But I think if he lives long enough, they'll be glad. When Matthew was in the unit, I was totally turned inward, I was almost autistic, nothing anyone could say would reach me. We had parents' group, and one day a woman came in and said her baby had been three months premature and that he had been on a ventilator and had a massive Grade 4 hemorrhage in his brain, and now he's happy and healthy. Just that little bit of hope changed everything. She wasn't telling me that my kid was going to be like that, but she was saying that he might, and it made such a big difference to me that I could bear to get close to Matthew."

Teresa's thoughts were so deeply in the past, her past, that it took her a moment to realize she was being asked a question. Kenny had looked at the crowded table in front of him and said, "I don't know if anyone in this room has a handicapped child . . ."

"I have a handicapped little boy," Teresa said. "His name is Matthew. He's a spastic quad," and she briefly explained her son's medical condition. "He goes to school, he's happy. To us, his life might be unacceptable, but to him it's all he knows, and he's happy."

For the first time since he began speaking, Kenny focused on one of the faces in the room. Claire, who had been staring at her folded hands, looked up and met Teresa's gaze. Everyone else at the table became a soft blur. All she saw was this one stranger who seemed to understand how she felt.

From then on, Kenny spoke directly to Teresa. His voice became animated where before it had been flat and somber.

"They say he'll never be able to move from here down," he said, placing the heel of his hand at his waist and sliding it toward his knees. "I don't believe that at all. I've seen him move his hips. I do hope he's not mentally handicapped because we're not going to be around all his life. I'd like to see him get a desk job, the kind of job I always wanted but never did get, where he sits at a desk and types in a machine maybe. Someplace clean."

"How do you feel about having a child with severe handicaps?" Sharon asked.

Kenny was startled. He had forgotten there were other people nearby.

"I feel we could deal with it."

He turned back toward Teresa. "We're not saying that because our son's not going to walk or ride a bicycle we're going to abandon him. We're going to do what's best for him, but if that means letting Landon go, then that is best."

"Do *you* think that's best?" Teresa asked. "Do *you* think you could do that?"

The couple had been in the room for nearly an hour, and Claire had not said a word. She sat watching her husband try to explain their feelings, and she grew steadily more angry. "Who are these people?" she thought. "Aren't they supposed to do the talking while we do the listening? Why are they making us defend our decision?

"The woman with the handicapped son is the only one who should be here. The rest of them are acting like they're judge and jury. What are we supposed to say? What do they want from us?

"None of the others has a handicapped child at home. They leave the hospital and go home to a perfectly normal happy world, so how can they possibly know? They go to school, and they read from books, and they know this and this about spina bifida, but do they know about trying to make a decision and live with it the rest of your life? About trying to decide whether you're going to let your child live, or let your child die?"

With these thoughts throbbing through her mind, Claire suddenly spoke her only sentence of the entire meeting. It came out with such force that she stunned the entire committee and even startled herself.

"I want to get out of here," she said.

Rattled and upset, Lin didn't try to change her mind.

"Thank you very much," she said to Claire, whom Kenny was already wheeling toward the door.

Once they were out of earshot, Lin put one hand to her burning stomach and said, "This is an ethical question that has no solution."

"Ethical questions by their very definition have no solutions," offered Dr. Van Eys.

"I think they were given too much information," said Dr. Oelberg, who had decided during the past hour that he would take this case back from José. "There are times when we ask parents to make the decisions. This should not be one of those times. I've pretty much made up my mind that I'm going to push them to do surgery. Not because I think it's the right thing to do, but because that's the easiest solution for these parents. I don't think there's going to be too much of a problem persuading. I hate to use that word because it sounds like I'm telling them what to do, but I think they will agree.

"But," he added, "that doesn't answer the real question, namely, 'Is it ethical not to operate?' I personally agree with Dr. Butler. If it were my child, I wouldn't operate. What I need to know is if they can't be persuaded, then does the committee think it's ethical to withhold surgery?"

"This committee member does," Margo Cox said. No one else spoke.

Doctors Butler, Oelberg, and Garcia left shortly thereafter, and the Ethics Committee set about the work of drafting its opinion. It took nearly thirty minutes—an eternity in medicine, where decisions are made and acted on every moment—to conclude that the surgery should be done. They never did agree, however, on *why* it should be done. Each member had a different reason for the conclusion, and not one of those reasons had very much to do with ethics.

Sharon believed surgery was the only approach that would keep the hospital out of court. Jim Grotta felt it was the only approach consistent with the committee's own guidelines. "I personally believe it's ethical not to operate," he said, "but I think our own rules say do it."

Listening to the half-hearted discussion, Randy struggled with the wording of the decision that would eventually find its way into Landon's chart.

"How would you like to phrase the question we're supposedly answering?" he asked.

"Is it ethical to withhold the standard of care?" Lin began to answer.

"I wouldn't use the term 'standard of care,'" Randy interrupted. "Not everyone agrees it is the standard of care."

"Is it ethical to allow the parents to refuse . . ." Jan Van Eys offered.

Randy interrupted again. "I would hate to memorialize the word 'refusal,'" he said.

He began to propose another approach. "Is it unethical to withhold . . ."

"I hate to use the word 'unethical,'" Dr. Van Eys said.

"How about 'appropriate'?"

"'Appropriate's' good."

Randy went back to scribbling and soon read aloud his final result:

"Ethical Issues: Whether surgical closure of the meningomyelocele should be done in light of the severity of the lesion and the father's wish that the child not be aggressively treated. Opinion: What needs to be considered in this opinion is whether the benefits of surgical closure outweigh the burdens incurred by the procedure. The procedure is palliative and will provide comfort to this baby. Therefore, the opinion of the IEC is that surgical closure is appropriate."

"That's waffling," Dr. Van Eys said when Randy finished reading.

"Yup," Randy said, "we waffled. But they waffled in our meeting. One waffle deserves another."

"I can't sign that," Dr. Cox said. "I'm sorry, but I think we're copping out."

Lin did not try to persuade her. "Does anyone else want their name taken off?" she asked.

No one answered, and the meeting was adjourned.

Patrick

When Patrick was wheeled back into the ICU after surgery, he was given a bed in the center of the room near the nurses' station. It was the spot he liked best in the place he hated most, but he was far too sick and medicated to notice. He had been given Pavulon, a paralyzing drug, so he would not fight the ventilator, and a large number of sedatives so he would not be aware of the temporary paralysis.

He paid no attention to the television set over his bed as the nurses flipped from the soap operas on ABC to the ones on CBS, then back again. He didn't see the name card placed at the foot of his bed, decorated with happy drawings of balloons, ice cream cones, and clowns, or the note Sally taped to the wall over his head warning: "Quiet! I am awake and can hear you. Please talk to me and not over me. Thanks, Patrick."

He was oblivious to the matter-of-fact approach to tragedy evident throughout the room: the file drawer labeled "Grief Support"; the desktop decorated with an aging copy of the Supportive Care Protocols. He was equally unaware of the constant presence of the nurses, who were eight hours into their twelve-hour shift when he arrived from the operating room at 3 P.M.

There was no question that the tiny body on the stretcher had been through a torturous ordeal. A bloodstained bandage nearly covered his entire chest, leaving a few scars from previous operations visible around the edges. His mouth was filled with a ribbed plastic tube that forked into a trident of smaller tubes, which in turn were hooked to the benign-looking box near the side of the bed labeled Servo Ventilator 900C. With each involuntary inhalation and exhalation, the tubes bobbed and vibrated.

Patrick's eyelids were taped down to keep his eyes from drying out. Two tubes had been forced into his nose and down his throat, one to drain secretions and the other to carry liquid nutrition to his stomach. Tubes were also held by needles in both his ankles, one bringing saline, the other bringing his bag of TPN. Yet another tube dangled from his right hand, at the ready to administer medication in a hurry. There was a separate line in his wrist allowing easy access to his veins when blood samples were required.

Two large tubes, which looked like garden hoses, snaked out of the side of his chest and were attached to a plastic, water-filled box. Bubbles percolated through the water as the tubes drew out air that was trapped in the chest during surgery. Electrical sensors were taped to his chest to measure his respiration rate and the heartbeat. A similar sensor was taped to his finger to measure the percentage of oxygen in his blood. Every tube and wire and machine had its own alarm system, and if any number fell too low or rose too high, there would be an attention-demanding ring, buzz, or beep.

He was examined by Dr. Andrassy and several surgical residents at 4 P.M., and appeared as stable as could be expected. At 4:30 he had some difficulty breathing. The attending doctor in the ICU ordered some changes in the settings on the ventilator, and that seemed to solve the problem. At five o'clock he began bleeding profusely, thoroughly soaking his bandages. Then, just as suddenly, the bleeding stopped. His blood pressure dropped chillingly low. The ICU staff theorized that he was bleeding into the sac around the heart, filling the sac with so much blood that there was no room for the heart to beat. If something dramatic wasn't done soon, Patrick would die.

Dr. Andrassy was paged and arrived at the ICU within minutes, wearing the green surgical scrubs in which he spends most of his day. The chief surgical resident was already at Patrick's side, as were the three pediatric residents, the ICU attending and four ICU nurses. Everyone was doing something. Nothing was working.

"How aggressive do we want to be?" Dr. Andrassy asked.

"He's DNR, but we just can't stand here."

"Is he DNR? I thought they changed that when they decided on surgery. What's the logic of operating on someone you're allowing to die?"

"A chest tube won't do it, he already has a chest tube," said the surgical resident. "If it's a tamponade, we have to go in and drain it."

"I don't think it's a tamponade, it's not that simple," Dr. Andrassy said.

"What then?"

"I think he's dying, of infection and everything that's gone on."

"We have to open him anyway, just to make sure. We can't have him dying of something we can fix."

"Let's do it."

With no time to transfer Patrick to an operating room, the two surgeons ripped off Patrick's bandages right there in the ICU, then sliced through the incision they had closed a few hours earlier and exposed Patrick's heart. Richard Andrassy can remember only a handful of times that he had to reopen a patient out of the operating room. The overused expression "A matter of life and death" applies literally on such occasions, and the adrenaline surge in the ears can be noisier than any ICU machine.

There was little time for anesthesia and, fortunately, there was no need. Deep blue sterile surgical drapes appeared as if from heaven, along with a medical staple remover designed to pull surgical staples from the skin with a crisp click. With the staples out, Patrick's skin parted easily, revealing the wires that held his rib cage in place. Two well-placed snips by Dr. Andrassy and the ribs yawned apart as well, exposing Patrick's beating heart.

There was some bleeding and fluid buildup. A syringe inserted into the cavity withdrew 100 ccs of liquid, enough to fill 6 tablespoons but not enough to cause Patrick's downward spiral.

"The blood's not the problem," Dr. Andrassy said. "I was hoping it was, but it's not. The real cause of the problem is Patrick, not the blood."

By 10:30 that night Patrick was once again considered stable. The next morning found him still paralyzed by his medication, but as the day wore on and the drugs wore off, he was awake sporadically and aware enough to follow a command to squeeze a nurse's hand. By evening he was writing notes to the staff. The ventilator tube and chest drainage tubes were removed the following morning, and he lay in his bed sucking on ice chips and asking for morphine.

It was midafternoon when he began to complain that his left leg wouldn't move. His left arm was numb too. "What's the deal with my leg?" he asked Javier.

"That will keep you from running around and causing trouble," joked Javier, avoiding the question. The paralysis could be temporary, but Javier didn't really think it was. In his opinion, a blood clot had broken off from the mass in Patrick's chest and traveled to the brain.

Paralysis was hardly Patrick's only problem. X rays showed that the newly inserted central line had slipped too far into the right ventricle of the heart, where it could potentially scramble the electrical system that regulates the heartbeat. Only another operation could correct the problem. He was still having breathing problems, his blood pressure was still low, and he was running a slight fever, evidence of an infection. Despite all this, he was ruled healthy enough to leave the ICU three days after surgery. With much fanfare, he was wheeled down the hall to his favorite pediatrics floor. Hours after he arrived, Javier entered a note in his chart: "Patrick is once again DNR."

Landon

Dr. José Garcia excused himself from the conference room across from Turner shortly after Claire and Kenny walked in.

"I'm sorry, I'm no longer on Landon's case," he told them as he offered a good-bye handshake. "There comes a time when you realize you're too close to a patient, and I think this is one of those times."

He had decided upon this emotional recusal a few hours earlier, at the meeting of the Ethics Committee. Listening to Kenny's anguish and confusion, he concluded that these parents needed a doctor they could see as impartial. They should feel they are making a decision between different options, not different doctors.

"Dr. Oelberg will be directing this meeting instead of me," he said, motioning toward David Oelberg, who had seated himself in one of the two straight-backed chairs. Dr. Hatem Megahed was seated in the other. That left the couch for Claire and Kenny. Meetings in this room were often choreographed that way: the doctors in the angular chairs, the patients in the soft, mushy couch.

Once the door had closed behind José, the two remaining doctors followed the script as they had prepared it with the committee. It was a short meeting, based on the premise that the surgery would in fact take place. That was fine with Kenny and Claire. Seeing Landon that morning, together, as a family, had made them reconsider surgery. They were exhausted and quite willing to have a doctor with a firm hand tell them what to do.

"You've already heard from three doctors that you can do one of two things," Dr. Oelberg said, ticking off the options from pinkie to thumb as he spoke. "These doctors aren't crazy, and they aren't incompetent. They're all very good doctors. They're disagreeing, and doctors will always disagree. So it's not that one is right and one is wrong. They're both right, depending upon what fits in with your family. There are plenty of babies who come through here with a meningomyelocele who can bring a lot of happiness to their parents. He's not going to play football. He may have problems at school from a cognitive point of view. But he may bring you just as much joy, if not more, than someone who starts out as a perfectly normal baby."

He paused, and then gave the persuasive push he had promised the Ethics Committee. "I would recommend that you repair it," he said. "If you feel otherwise, I'm willing to consider that, but I recommend you repair it. Otherwise I'm afraid you'll spend your life wishing that you had."

Dr. Megahed nodded. "I feel like your baby has a chance," he said. "I think we should take that chance."

Kenny looked at Claire, then at David Oelberg. For a moment Dr. Oelberg thought the young father was about to disagree. But when Kenny spoke, he said only a single word: "When?"

"In a day or two," Dr. Oelberg said. "Does that mean you've decided?"

"I think we've finally decided," said Claire.

"Finally," said Kenny.

The surgery took place the following day.

Patrick

The first order of business upon Patrick's return to the pediatric unit was his room assignment. He asked for the room closest to the nurses' station, the one with a plaque on the door that reads, "Care by Parent. Furnishings by Houston Chapter, Jane Phillips Sorority, 1977." Fortunately, the room was available. No one wanted to say no to Patrick.

Before long he was fully settled in the familiar surroundings of Room 3431. A hand-lettered sign, the handiwork of one of the nurses, joined the bronze one on the door: "Please leave the door half opened when no one is with patient. Thank you. Pat and the management."

The second order of business was what to do about the fact that the newly inserted central line had apparently slipped too far into the heart. For two days Patrick's doctors communicated by chart, all coming to the same conclusion. "Given the extreme high risk of reoperation, we will opt to leave the catheter position as is permanently," Dr. Andrassy wrote.

"I would accept the risk of arrhythmias when compared to a possible surgical reintervention," Javier wrote. "The risk of returning Patrick to surgery is much greater than that of leaving the catheter in place." He left his deepest thoughts unwritten: "At this point, if he has a sudden death, it will be a blessing."

The third bit of business was not so easily solved. With each day it became more certain that Patrick was paralyzed on his left side. He could feel sensation in his left arm and leg, but he couldn't make either of those limbs move. He could shrug his shoulder a little, but he couldn't bend his wrist or elbow. He could flex his fingers slightly, but he couldn't touch his forefinger to his thumb.

It was unclear what had caused the paralysis. At first, Javier's assumption was that a blood clot had broken loose after surgery and been swept through the bloodstream and into the brain. But CAT scans of Patrick's head a few days later showed no sign of such a clot, leading Javier to believe that a clump of yeast from someplace in Patrick's infected body had broken off and lodged in the brain. It would have done the same damage as a vagrant clot, but would have left no mark on a CAT scan. This was only a theory. Javier had no way to confirm it and no way to reverse the effects.

Mary Coffey and the others in the Occupational Therapy Department did what little they could to help. Patrick's left hand was placed in a splint to keep the fingers curved slightly in a functioning position just in case movement ever returned. He was also taught a series of exercises he could do himself, using his right arm to lift and bend his left leg.

He rebelled stubbornly against his newest limitations, refusing, for instance, to use his bedpan, and insisting on getting out of bed in order to use the toilet. He never made it. Each time he tried, he would crash to the floor, and a nurse would have to come and lift him onto the toilet and then into bed. This mortified him, but not enough to keep him from trying the same stunt again and again.

After several failed attempts, Kay marched in with a look on her face that Patrick knew meant business.

"Listen," she said, with her hands on her hips in her best disciplinarian tone. "You do *not* get up without somebody in here. We'll respect your privacy. We'll leave once we know you're safe. We'll stand outside the door. We won't stay in here while you're on the pot, but you *have* to get someone."

Patrick was lying on his bed, his back propped against pillows, his good leg bent under him and his bad leg out straight. He stared at Kay while she spoke. When she stopped talking, she expected him to argue with what she had said. He surprised her.

"You never told me I'd be paralyzed," he said in a tone of quiet accusation.

Nothing he could have said could have hurt Kay more.

"I didn't know."

"Well, you *should* have known. You should have told me. You told me I might die, but you didn't tell me about this."

"I didn't know, Patrick. Really, I didn't know."

Over the next few days Patrick seemed to decide that his condition was temporary, asking, "When can I go back to school? When can I walk to school? When can I go home?"

Javier tried to encourage the optimism without telling any outright lies. "When we send you home, I'll throw you a big party at my house," he said. "Start working on the guest list."

Javier feared it would be a very long time before he would host such a party. The new line was working well, but very little else in Patrick's body was functioning properly. He was always tired and breathless, and he ran a fever constantly. Every day he had at least one period when he simply couldn't breathe. In part, that was due to the buildup of fluid in his chest, a result of infection, surgery, and a possible embolism in his lungs, similar to the one that probably entered his brain and caused his paralysis. In part, however, it was more complicated than that. The new central line was, as feared, meddling with the electrical current of his heart and causing what he called "the funny feelings," much like palpitations. The funny feelings, in turn, made him feel as if he couldn't breathe. The one thing Patrick feared most was not being able to breathe. It was why he refused to lie down in the operating room: The anesthesia mask on his face made him feel like he was being suffocated. So at the first hint of these catheter-induced chest pains, Patrick would panic. The more anxious he became, the more difficult it was for him to breathe, and soon his fear of suffocation began to turn real.

"I can't breathe, sit me up," he'd yell from his bed. The nurses would give him oxygen through a face mask and prop him with pillows until he was sitting ramrod straight, but it wasn't enough to calm him.

"Sit me up, sit me up."

"Patrick, you are up."

"Then give me oxygen."

"Your oxygen's on."

"I can't breathe, I can't breathe."

To combat these episodes, Javier ordered a diuretic to flush the excess fluid from Patrick's lungs, and liberal doses of Ativan and morphine to calm him. That worked only some of the time. Even between these breathing episodes, Patrick was anxious. Periodically, he would ring the buzzer by his bed to summon the nurses. "I'm scared," he would tell them.

"Of what?"

He never answered.

"Let me know if you want to talk."

Minutes to hours later he would ring again.

His obvious fear of dying and his reluctance to raise the issue reopened the debate on the pediatric floor over whether someone should talk to Patrick about death. It also gave new urgency to the question of what more should be done to keep the boy from dying. Javier, unwilling to make a decision on his own, called two meetings. At 1 P.M. he met with the doctors and therapists who worked regularly with Patrick. Two hours later, he met with most of the pediatric nursing staff. Although he called the meetings out of a need for guidance, it turned out that he did most of the talking, saying much the same thing at both meetings. Tears flowed freely from the speaker and his listeners.

"There will be no more surgeries," he said. "I will not offer him that option again. I could not talk to him the way I did ten days ago and say, 'Look, these are your options.' There is no option anymore.

"Our main priority now is comfort," he continued, "and to make it possible for him to go home. He is now on Supportive Protocol Two. He will not be resuscitated. If he needs oxygen, we will give him as much as he needs. If he is anxious, we will give him morphine. But he will not be resuscitated. I hope I can be there."

"Do we tell all this to Patrick?" Kay asked. She put the question to Javier only because so many of her nurses had put it to her in recent days. Personally, she had become comfortable abiding by Oria's wishes. She would not bring the subject up unless Patrick did. He wanted to die, she was certain of that, and she believed that, if he knew the meaning of Supportive Protocols and DNR, he would ask for it. He had learned what "doing everything" means in modern medicine, and he'd had enough.

"We'll answer his questions, but that's all," Javier said, remembering his promise to Oria, too.

"What about the ampho?" Richard asked at the first meeting.

"Let's not discontinue it yet. It's still keeping the infection under control."

"Lord, I hope he doesn't die on my shift," one of the nurses said at the second meeting.

Quickly Javier shook his head to clear the deathbed scene that was forming with eerie clarity in his mind.

"I would like to send him home next week," he said. "I'd also like to try increasing his medication. The Ativan keeps him calm, but it wears off before twelve hours, so I think he should have it more than that. Don't worry about addicting him. That's the least of his problems."

The nurses began to list what Patrick would need if he were to be sent home.

"His grandmother's house is the logical place, since Mom's never home."

"He'll need a wheelchair, a potty chair, oxygen, morphine."

With the increase in his medication, Patrick seemed to improve. He was less anxious, his gasping spells were less frequent, he seemed to be in less pain, he even did the exercises for his left arm and leg. Two days after the meetings of the staff, Patrick announced to Javier, "I want to go home today."

"You're not quite ready," Javier said, pleased by the demand. He made a deal with Patrick. Instead of a discharge home, Javier would authorize a pass allowing Patrick and Oria to leave the hospital the following day. He could use it to go wherever he wished.

"I want to see the Blue Angels," Patrick said, naming a stunt flying show that was in town for several days. That week, Patrick had decided he wanted to be a pilot when he grew up.

Patrick

The Blue Angels air show was as exciting as Patrick had imagined. But he wasn't there to watch. He spent the entire day in his bed at Hermann, too ill to use the precious one-day pass. The following morning he opened his eyes to find the Blue Angels themselves standing by his bed, the speedy result of Richard's call to the Make-A-Wish foundation. Patrick shook their hands and accepted their honorary membership pin, but he barely smiled.

Kay began to fear that he would never smile again. In the days after the stunt pilots' visit, he became steadily more withdrawn, refusing to talk or leave his room. One morning he asked for a needle and syringe, saying he needed to flush out his central line. The nurses refused, and that evening he was caught rummaging frantically through the needle box in his room.

"I want a needle to stick in my line so I can die," he said, once the box was grabbed from him. "I hurt all over. I want it to stop."

He started to cry, and he kept crying most of the night. He was still crying when Javier came to see him early in the morning. "I don't want to be this way. I want to go home. I want this to stop," he said.

The door to his room was kept open all day and all night, and a nurse stopped to see him at least twice an hour. Near dawn, he had another of his suffocating spells, the worst one so far. "The Lasix didn't work, neither did the morphine," Kay told Javier. "Nothing was touching it. Nothing."

"I think we should stop the ampho," Javier said. He believed that the side effects of the toxic drug were compounding Patrick's pain and discomfort, and he could no longer justify their use. "We're not curing him of the infection, we're making him miserable," he said. "The cure would have been a long time ago. The cure would have been to get the catheter out."

Finally, Javier had made the decision. Let Patrick die. Let the infection kill him.

"Due to persistent infection, the multiple side effects of the amphotericin, and being unable to clear the infection we will *stop* the amphotericin," he wrote in Patrick's chart. "He will *not* be treated for any additional infection, he will not be intubated, no CPR effort will be started and there is no indication to transfer him to the PCCU."

No one told Patrick that he would no longer be receiving his amphotericin. No one told him how close he was to death. But on the day the ampho was stopped, Patrick began to say good-bye to the staff. One by one, he called his favorite, and not so favorite, nurses and doctors to his room and made childlike peace.

"Thank you for helping me and my mother," he told Sally. She took his hand in hers and squeezed it, hard. He squeezed back. With that gesture Sally felt she had been allowed into his circle. It made her feel she had the right to grieve at his imminent death as a friend instead of as an outsider.

Oria also noticed a difference in her son. "He's so sweet today," she said after her brief afternoon visit. She was on her way home to run some errands, she said, but she planned to return later and sleep in Patrick's room all night.

Near midnight, Christine Gladden, who had been his nurse for five years, left his room near tears. "He said, 'I want to tell you all I love you very much,' " she said. "He was saying it to me, but he was really saying it to everyone. He said, 'I want to thank you for all you've done for me. I'm real tired now and I want to go to sleep.' "

At 1:45 A.M., the resident on call was paged to Patrick's bedside. The unconscious boy could not breathe. His nostrils were flaring with the effort and his chest wall caved inward with each labored breath. The monitor that measured the level of oxygen in his blood gave a piercing, shrieking beep. Normal levels are between 95 and 100. Patrick's was in the 80s before the resident even arrived. A face mask was slammed over Patrick's mouth and an aerosol dose of Vaponefrin, designed to open tightened air passages, was administered. The monitor dropped into the 70s. Thirty milligrams of Lasix, which reduces fluid buildup, was injected into the IV. The monitor dropped to 66. His heart rate was 150 beats per minute, incredibly fast.

"Administer oxygen and call his mother," the resident said.

Oria was home doing an overwhelming pile of laundry when the telephone rang.

"I'll be there soon," she said.

"I think you should get here now."

By the time she arrived, Patrick's gasping and flailing had stopped. He lay in his bed with his eyes closed, breathing very, very slowly. She knew he was alive because there were hills and valleys on his monitors, but his breathing was so shallow that she found herself holding her own breath while waiting for his chest to rise and fall.

The night staff let her be alone with him, though they came in every few minutes to record numbers off the machines. At 3 A.M., one of the nurses called Kay. She got up and took a shower before driving through the blackness to the hospital. She knew it would be a long, grueling day.

Kay walked into Patrick's room an hour later. His oxygen saturation level was at 20 percent. Oria was lying in bed next to Patrick, cradling him with one arm and running her fingers through his matted, sweat-drenched hair. Kay said nothing, not wanting to leave, but not wanting to interrupt. Without warning there was a loud beep from the assorted machines by the bed. Patrick had stopped breathing. For a moment Kay fought the urge to *do* something: start CPR, inject a drug. It was instinct. But it passed. This was right. It was time.

Oria sat upright with a jolt. Panicked, she reached for the emergency call button at the side of the bed and frantically pressed it. She looked across her son's body and saw Kay for the first time.

"Our baby is dead," she wailed. "Kay, our baby is dead, our baby is dead, our baby is dead."

Patrick Dismuke was pronounced dead at 4:45 A.M. on October 7, 1988. Sally Olsen's grandfather clock stopped at exactly that time. Javier Aceves was notified immediately.

"Called by Dr. Wiseman about Patrick's death," he wrote as his final entry in the chart. "Patrick's body looks relaxed. In peace. The most likely cause of death was a pulmonary embolism. Autopsy was refused."

Epilogue

This book is about making choices—and living with them. As I write this, it has been nearly four years since most of these choices were made, enough time for the consequences to become clearer.

Armando Dimas believes he chose well, although he has had more than one chance to question his decision. Completely paralyzed and dependent on a ventilator, he was sent to live at Bart's, which came to feel like home. His room there was decorated with bright animal posters and pictures of his family. His parents came to visit every weekend, bringing his son, Armando, Jr., who had moved in with them in Madisonville.

One thing Armando did not bring with him to Bart's was his specially ordered wheelchair. It arrived at Hermann shortly before he left for Bart's and, despite Mary Coffey's careful planning, it was too big. His body fit better than it had in any of the chairs that Hermann owned, but his head still slipped uncomfortably from side to side. Mary cobbled a headpiece with parts scavenged from a storeroom, but the result was less than perfect, and she always brought a toolbox to his exercise sessions just in case the chair needed repair. When Armando was transferred from Hermann, the rented wheelchair was left behind, and an acceptable model was found for him in Bart's storeroom.

Armando found a kind of peace at Bart's. Every so often someone would ask him if he wanted to be made DNR, and he would always say no. One afternoon I went to visit and asked that question myself. "If you get very sick," I said, "do you want them to try to make you better or do you want them to let you die?"

He looked confused.

"I want them to make me better," he said.

"The reason I ask," I said, "is that a lot of people would look at you and think they wouldn't want to live like that."

"I see my family," he answered. "My sister brings me food. It's nice here." Unable to point, he wrinkled his sunburned nose, a result of the morning he spent sitting in the courtyard of Bart's. "See, I go outside a lot," he said. "In a lot of ways, things are good."

He paused, trying to explain the gritty life he had led before and how the accident and its aftermath had changed everything. "If I hadn't been shot," he said, "I would have died."

Just weeks later, however, Armando found himself angrily asking to die. The cost of his care had increased steadily during his years at Bart's, and the financial office at Hermann Hospital decided it simply could not pay his bills for the rest of his life. Money was not the only reason for their decision, the hospital said. It was better for a patient to be with his family, and it was time to send Armando home.

Without money from Hermann, Bart's could not afford to let him stay. One morning the Dimas family came to visit and were informed that Armando had to leave.

"Where can I go?" he asked forlornly, when his mother told him the news. "Why don't they just wheel me out to the sidewalk and let me die?"

Hermann gave Bart's one month to train the family to care for Armando, and all his brothers, sisters, their spouses and children took lessons in how to lift, feed, wash, change, position, and suction him. During years of visits to Bart's, the Dimas family found the machines less intimidating and his routines more familiar, but it was still far from clear that they could learn all there was to know about how to keep Armando comfortable and alive.

His parents feared they could not handle the job alone, and moved twenty miles from Madisonville to Huntsville, where most of their children had settled and where there were more available hands. The stress took its toll on Victoria Dimas, who was hospitalized twice in the days before her son's return, because she was having trouble breathing.

On Halloween morning, 1992, an ambulance drove Armando home. He was frightened during the first few nights, certain that the electricity would fail and he would suffocate, since the family could not afford an emergency generator. Only a battery pack or a hand-operated pump would keep his ventilator working until power was restored.

But a call to the utility company brought assurances that he would not be left to die during a blackout. He feels safer now, secure in the fact that a member of his family is at his side every moment. His mother takes the day shift, two of his brothers alternate on the night shift, and everyone else helps when they can.

He is happy at home, he says. It's good to have his son nearby, and he is resigned to the fact that Hermann's promise to care for him had an expiration date.

"I was angry, but I'm less angry," he said two weeks

after he moved back home. "Things changed. This is the way it is. That's all."

Fran and Carey Poarch also believed they chose well—most of the time. One month after Taylor's death, Fran was pregnant again. Carey Poarch, Jr., was born healthy and without complications the following summer. His sister, Lucy, was born two years later.

Fran and Carey often tell their young children about the fragile babies who came first, and now and then the whole family visits the cemetery together. Someday, when the children are older, Fran and Carey plan to show them Taylor's hospital ID bracelet, which Fran still carries in her wallet.

Watching their healthy children grow, Fran and Carey are increasingly certain they were right to let Taylor die. But once in a while, in the middle of the night, there are doubts. I sent the Poarches an early draft of their story to read. Two days later my telephone rang at 2:30 A.M. It was Carey, and his voice was shaking.

"Did we do the wrong thing?" he asked, over and over. "I didn't know her eyes were open when they turned off the vent. Did we do the wrong thing?"

I reminded him that Lin Weeks had been sorry he and Fran had chosen not to attend the Ethics Committee meeting about Taylor. Lin believed that sometime in the future Fran and Carey would be comforted by the mental picture of a round table of doctors saying, "We agree with you."

"I was there, Carey," I said. "They were on your side."

"You have a baby. Do you think we did the right thing?" he asked.

"Yes," I said. "I do."

* * *

Claire and Kenny Sparks think about their decision every day. Landon is not doing well. For nearly two years he did very well—though confined to a wheelchair, he could see, hear, and talk. He loved music and games, and he had an infectious, happy laugh.

He needed constant physical therapy, however, and was prone to a variety of infections, particularly in his lungs, a side effect of not being able to move on his own. One day he developed bronchitis, and his fever rose to 105 degrees. At 3 A.M. his parents awoke to find him in the middle of a thrashing seizure, and within hours he was in Hermann Hospital on a ventilator.

Kenny and Claire wanted the machine disconnected. They had voted for life once before; this time they sought the peace of death. Landon's doctors suggested a meeting of the Ethics Committee, but Kenny and Claire refused to attend, remembering their awkwardness and rage the first time around. So the doctors eventually agreed that the ventilator could be removed. But when the machine was turned off, the little boy continued to breathe on his own.

He is back home now, in the trailer where he has lived all his life. He shares that home with his baby brother, Jared, who was born six months after his seizure. The Sparkses were shocked to learn that Claire was pregnant with Jared since it had taken the help of doctors and fertility drugs to conceive Landon. Now that Landon is back home, Claire tries not to resent her younger son for surpassing her older one. Kenny tries not to dwell on the guilt he feels that he didn't take Landon to the emergency room when the boy's fever began to rise.

The Sparkses don't go out much. Money is tight—most of it goes to pay Landon's medical bills—and there are few baby-sitters who want to stay with an unresponsive four-year-old. Landon has developed bed-sores on his back, which make it nearly impossible to put him in his car seat and take him out of the house. It has been a long time since Claire has gone anyplace other than the doctor, the children's school, her local church, or the Baytown mall.

Claire and Kenny often replay the choice they were given when Landon was born, with some doctors stressing the future and others stressing the moment.

"Would you make the same decision again?" I asked hesitantly during one particularly sad telephone call.

"I love him. I wouldn't trade him for anything," Claire said.

She sounded exhausted.

Every so often, Teresa Knepper runs into Claire, Kenny, Landon, and Jared at the mall. She comes away from those chance encounters deeply troubled. No longer a member of the Ethics Committee—the monthly meeting time was changed from Friday afternoons to Tuesday mornings, and she couldn't take that time slot off from work—the Sparks case is the one that she cannot forget.

Her own son is thriving at school, and she wonders whether the advice she gave the Sparkses at the Ethics Committee meeting—advice that encouraged them to save their son—was too optimistic.

"It's so sad," she said of Landon. "You look into his eyes, and you can almost see an unhappy little boy trying to get out."

Lin Weeks is no longer chairman of the Ethics Committee. She simply ran out of time and enthusiasm for her favorite project. Her job has become steadily more demanding every year, and most recently she was made vice-president of operations for Hermann, meaning that her already hectic schedule became unbearable.

"It got to the point where someone would call to ask for an Ethics Committee consult, and I would try to talk them out of it because I was too busy," she explained.

More has changed than just her schedule. She completed her Ph.D. and self-consciously uses the title "Dr." Her office is no longer a tiny box with an even tinier table. When I last visited, she and her new secretary shared a two room suite, complete with a private rest room.

She is, she said, more comfortable at Hermann than she was during her first few years as chairman of the Ethics Committee. "For a long time I was on the outside looking in," she said. "Now I'm definitely on the inside."

Hermann Hospital is in better financial health—the result of sharp cutbacks and shrewd marketing. When Patrick, Taylor, Armando, and Landon were there, the hospital was having a problem filling its beds. Now, Lin spends much of her time trying to find empty beds for the crush of patients.

In what has become a distressingly familiar scenario at Hermann, a new scandal resulted in the resignation of two members of the board of trustees of the Hermann Hospital Trust. Both board members were closely linked to a food distribution company that was extremely strapped for cash. The president of Hermann Hospital purchased nearly 100,000 pounds of fajita meat and smoked turkey from the company, saying the food was to be used for future hospital needs.

The $245,000 cost of meat was more than twice the limit on what the president was authorized to spend without prior approval. Most of the meat had not been delivered more than two months after it had been ordered. The meat that was delivered was used to fete the board and the staff, not to feed the patients. These facts combined to raise the question of whether the transaction was really a purchase at all, or whether it was a way for the hospital to provide a fast, interest-free loan to a company whose chairman and attorney were also trustees of the Hermann Trust.

The entire episode has become known as Fajitagate. The president was fired. He subsequently passed a lie detector test. The two trustees in question resigned. About a month after the story broke, a group of former employees of Hermann gathered at a Mexican restaurant for a reunion. All had been laid off from Hermann because of budget cuts. The menu for the reunion party: fajitas.

Oria Dismuke left Hermann, but not because of budget cuts. She felt lost for more than a year after Patrick died, and she was fired from her job in the Hermann cafeteria for chronic tardiness. Now she thinks she was being late "almost on purpose" because she couldn't bear to go inside the hospital.

We met for a soda and a quick hello recently, and she looked downright happy—an expression I hadn't seen during the entire time I'd known her. She was in love, she explained, with a man she had worked with at Hermann. He was kind to her after Patrick's death, and she is grateful to him for that kindness. They keep meaning to get married, she said, they just haven't found the time. She has a new job—as a cashier at a local Shell service station. Things are busy, she said, but she would take a vacation soon and make it her honeymoon.

I read her the parts of this book that were about her

and her son. "I was bone tired then," she said, when I'd finished. "I wasn't a bad mother. They thought I didn't care sometimes, but they didn't understand. I was tired. He was sick fifteen years. We both were tired."

Javier left Hermann, and Sally followed soon after. She went to head the pediatric clinic at a small San Antonio hospital. He went to run the pediatric service at a tiny hospital in Albuquerque devoted entirely to handicapped children. He has pictures of Patrick in his office.

In the months after Patrick's death, Javier thought about becoming an administrator or maybe a professor—anything that would give him needed distance from his patients. He enrolled in courses on medical ethics. He shaved his mustache to create a symbolic clean slate.

The job offer in Albuquerque provided a perfect opportunity to start over. Mostly he took the position for his children. Paco had been in remission for five years—the medical definition of cured—and the family no longer had to cling to Houston in fear that their boy would fall sick again. But he also moved because of Patrick.

"I wasn't really burned out," he said, after he, Roseanne, and the children were settled in their new home. "But I needed a change."

His brief doubts that he could care for patients again are gone. He sees sick children four days a week in the hospital clinic, and every Friday he flies to small towns all over New Mexico to visit patients who cannot come to him.

"Now I look back on that time as a time of struggle, of growing pains," he said of the last months of Patrick's life. "I was right out of my residency, and I wasn't ready to handle it.

"I still wonder whether I looked at all the possibilities to help him," he said, "but I don't live hurting. Maybe I've finally learned how to protect myself."

Acknowledgments

This book is the result of the nearly three years I spent with the Ethics Committee of Hermann Hospital in Houston, Texas, beginning in May of 1988. During that time, I attended the committee's meetings, interviewed its members, and watched as doctors and patients made decisions about life and death.

This is a work of nonfiction, and everything—to the best of my knowledge—is true. The events chronicled here all took place between May and October of 1988, although some of the explanatory anecdotes occurred in subsequent months. I observed many of the events and conversations firsthand, and when I was not present, I relied on the description of at least one person who was there. To ensure that my words matched their memories, I asked nearly all the participants to read the pages that told their stories before the book went to print.

Because this is nonfiction, I wanted all the names to be real. Nearly everyone interviewed for the book agreed that I could use their names, with four exceptions: the families of Mr. Hardy, Mrs. Fence, and Dexter Advani, and nurse Virginia Lennox. Those names are my creations although their stories are true. All the other names are real.

Lin Weeks, former chairman of the Ethics Committee, used time she did not have to guide me through questions of medical ethics in general and the workings of her committee in particular. I could not have written this book without her.

Similarly, Christine LeLaurin, formerly of Hermann's public relations staff, parted the bureaucracy for me because she felt the subject was important. She provided me with an official hospital ID badge, my own parking card, and permission to roam freely about the hospital. She also provided a wellspring of knowledge about Hermann.

A long list of people invited me into their lives during the course of my research. I admire them for the courage they showed in the shadow of tragedy, and their generosity in allowing me to share some very personal moments and memories. To Oria Dismuke, Fran and Carey Poarch, Armando Dimas, and Claire and Kenny Sparks, I want to say Thank You. I hope my constant prodding and questioning didn't cause you any additional pain.

Thank you, too, to the doctors whose lives intersected with these patients, and who were equally generous with their thoughts and their time. Javier Aceves, Kay Tittle, Sally Olsen, Sharon Crandell, Teresa Knepper, and Cindy Walker were people I looked to particularly often for advice. And Stanley J. Reiser and Jan Van Eys require special mention because, I'm afraid, the hours they spent educating me are not properly represented in the book.

While researching and writing this book, I found the work of countless other authors to be enlightening and thought-provoking. Among those upon whom I relied most are the following: *The Social Transformation of Medicine*, by Paul Starr; *Strangers at the Bedside*, by David J. Rothman; *What Kind of Life* and *Setting Limits*, both by Daniel Callahan; *Institutional Ethics Com-*

mittees and Health Care Decision Making, edited by Ronald E. Cranford and A. Edward Doudera; *Mortal Choices*, by Ruth Macklin; and Harry Hurt III's chronicle of Hermann Hospital for *Texas Monthly*.

My other, "real-life," job is as a reporter for *The New York Times*, and my colleagues in the Houston bureau of that paper were kind enough to help me juggle both the book and the news: Peter Appleborne, Roberto Suro, Maureen Balleza, Linda Barth, Ann Wozencraft, and Maria Moss. Soma Golden, the national editor of the *Times*, showed great faith by helping me find a place in the Houston bureau. Jon Landman and Peter Kaufman made me look good while I was in Texas, and taught me how indispensable good editing can be.

And speaking of good editing, Esther Fein has the sharp pen of a gifted writer and the soft touch of a dear friend. Bob Asahina of Simon & Schuster gently suggested, dissected, rejiggered, and buffed—and kindly allowed me to believe I was doing it all myself. His help was surpassed only by that of Kathy Robbins of the Robbins office. Every author should have an agent this perfect.

I was lucky enough to have relatives who are also experts in medicine, science, law, and public health: my parents, Myron and Janet Belkin; my siblings, Gary Belkin and Kira Belkin; Noemi and Allen Gelb; Alan Safran and Dana Gelb Safran; and Masha Schiller Belkin.

Thanks also to Susan Chira, who reads every word, as did Sharon Hall and Todd Kessler. Elizabeth Barnes, Barbara Laing, Chris Keyser, David Sanger, Mimi Swartz, Jeff and Patti Towbin, and Lisa Wolfe were always willing to listen. And I owe an overdue apology to David Morris and Susan Farb Morris, who happened to ask how it was going one day when it wasn't going particularly well.

Finally, this book is dedicated to three people who shape my view of life and whose influence is found throughout these pages.

My husband, Bruce Gelb, is the best doctor I know, my private example of how skill can mesh seamlessly with compassion.

My son, Evan Phillip, was born halfway through the book's second draft. He made the whole world seem new, and the idea of a child in pain seem unbearable.

My grandmother Pearl Ehrenreich died before this book was completed. She brought dignity to her life and her death. I hope she would have been proud.